I0828279

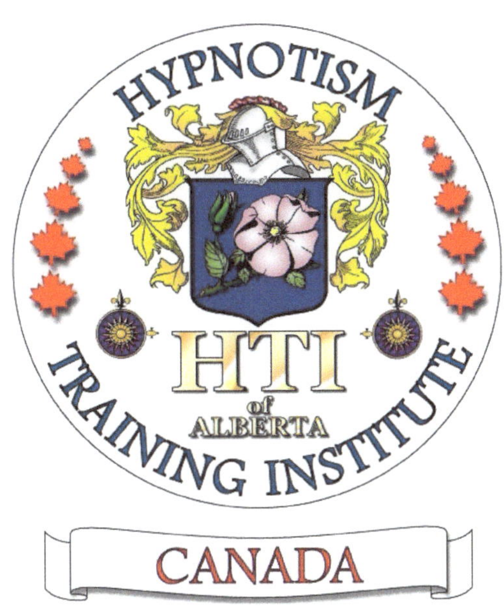

Hypnosis 602

Physiological Stress Release

By Anny J. Slegten

Physiological Stress Release
Anny Slegten
Published by
Kimberlite Publishing House
www.kimberlitePublishingHouse.com

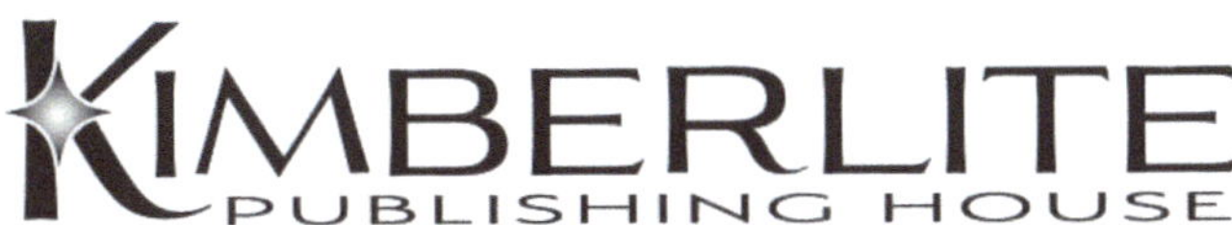

The author of this book does not dispense medical advice or prescribe the use of any technique as a form of treatment for physical, emotional, mental, spiritual or medical problems without the advice of a physician, either directly or indirectly. The intent of the author is only to offer information of a general nature to help you in your quest for physical, mental, emotional and spiritual wellbeing.

In the event you use any of the information in this book for yourself, which is your right, the author and the publisher assume no responsibility for your actions.

ISBN: 978-1-7775332-0-5

School Coat of Arms designed by Boomer Stralak
Book layout by Colin Christopher *www.colinchristopher.com*
Book cover and Kimberlite Logo designed by Marietta Miller
www.execugraphx.com

The Kimberlite-Diamond Connection

Kimberlite is a rock type that was first categorized over a 100 years ago based on descriptions of the diamond-bearing pipes of Kimberley, South Africa.

Kimberlites are the mechanism by which diamonds are brought to the surface.

Kimberlitic rocks are the most important primary source of diamonds and the main rock type in which significant diamond deposits have been found so far.

Anny is familiar with many rocks and minerals as her husband was raised around quarries, and later worked in several mines in Canada.

Therefore, it was natural for Anny to choose kimberlite as an analogy to the soul residing within our body – as a diamond within the kimberlite.

A Picture Is Worth A Thousand Words – The Bird Bath

From the house veranda, I enjoy watching birds frolicking in the bird bath, ruffling their feathers, and picking out whatever they feel should not be hiding there.

They then get out of the water, stand at the hedge of the bird bath, give themselves a good shake and happily fly off to resume the duty of the day.

Just like us, allowing our soul, out diamond as I call it, to feel cleaner and shine in its full beauty each time we resolve an issue weighting on our conscious, bringing with it a much-needed peace of mind.

As you know by now, our soul chose a physical life to speed up evolving our soul, having resolved what weighs heavily in our conscious.

By being true to ourselves, resolving issues now, we are hopefully preparing ourselves for a better life after this physical one.

With Love and Light,

Anny.

Welcome to

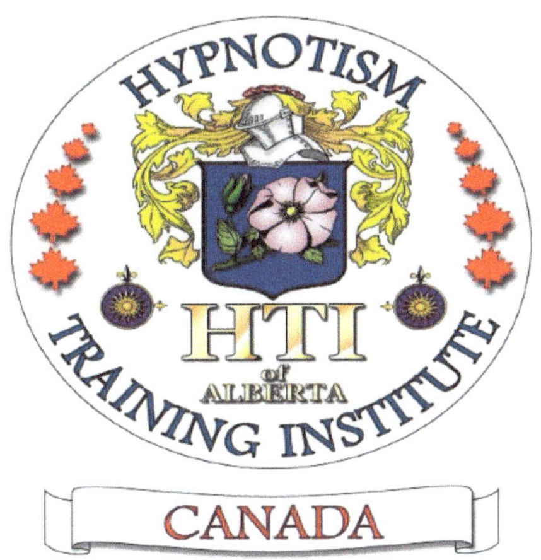

HYP 602 – Physiological Stress Release

This book belongs to:

Name ______________________________

Mailing Address ______________________________

____

City or Town ______________________________

Province/State ____________________ Postal Code/Zip ________

Country ______________________________

Telephone Home (___) __________ Work (___) __________

Instructor's Name: ***Anny Slegten***

Today's Date: ______________________________

Foreword

This Is All About The Soma, Or Is It?

HYP 602 - Physiological Stress Release

***Prerequisite: HYP 101, 201, 202, 203, 204 and HYP 601.**

This course is all about the Soma, the physical body, and the skill of accessing the etheric body to obtain what is going on at subconscious level and expresses itself in the physical body.
At the end of this course, you will realize how true it is that our physical body is dependent of how we think and feel.

Yes, Energy is Everything and Everything is Energy.

The Workshop (presented in 5 parts)

1) Hypnosis in the Field - for emergencies and emergency medical responders

2) Body Cell Regression

The Question

Is it possible to take control over genetics, and limitations placed on us by our ancestors? Can these limitations be the residues of physical and emotional traumas manifesting in various physical and emotional disorders?

Answer

Profound emotions are 'frozen' in the cells (genetic memory) and passed on from generation to generation. For this technique, the client goes down the family tree, accessing ancestral memories, to unlock the cause of the "family curse". The intentions are to free future generations from these limitations, as well restoring physical equilibrium to the present generation, allowing the body to enjoy perfect harmony as presently intended.

3) Emotional Stress Release

The Question

Can a harmonious bond between the psyche and the soma be restored, allowing the body to enjoy perfect harmony as presently intended?

Answer

Emotional Stress Release can be effective in many situations, including in cases of discovering the impact of a highly emotional event, frozen in the body.
After an accident or traumatic event, "chronic pain" can be manifestations of emotional issues (it becomes evident when after exhausting all physical resources, a person is told "it's all in the head". Counseling techniques on the trigger and releasing of these issues will be demonstrated. The technique is simple, compassionate, and usually restores emotional order in one session.

4) Physical Stress Release

The Technique

The client is first lead into a hypnotic trance, and then encouraged to access and trigger the memories of the trauma by acknowledging a physical discomfort. As stated before, this technique is as efficient as it is simple. The information comes spontaneously and with great emotion. There will be demonstrations followed by practice sessions.

5) Accessing what is going inside, affecting the outside, the physical body.

This part is about 'reading' a person, an animal or even energy field of anything that exist.

There are many techniques to do so, including 'reading' a person's or animal's energy field to know where the body hurts … if any (!) as well as how the physical body responds to street drugs and medication.

The Results

With emotional order comes clear memory and an awakening of the body. Consequently, some clients have experienced total feeling back in their limbs; total freedom from allergies; complete release of chronic pain; to just mention a few cases. Remember, the technique being demonstrated is not meant as a substitute for medical or psychological help. Instead it is a powerful adjunct.

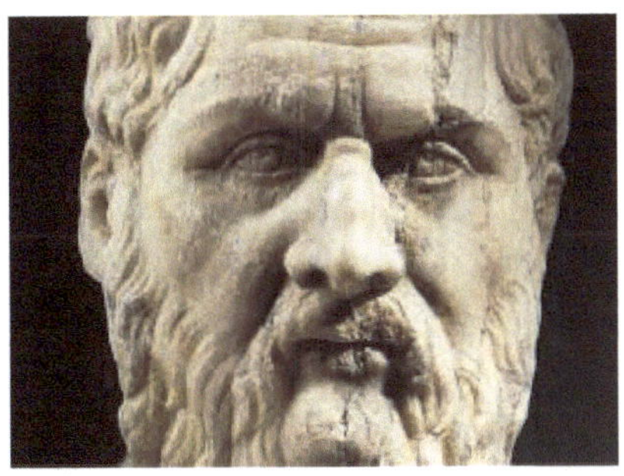

To quote Plato 428 – 348 BC

To heal the body, you must first heal the mind

Table Of Contents

A Note From Anny

The design and development of the Course Material required the investment of substantial effort, time and money and is only intended for the participants of HYP 602, Physiological Stress Release.

Understand that the experiences derived from attending this course is a private and personal experience for each participant. As such please do respect the confidentiality of all participants and their remarks and actions and keep all such information private and confidential.

As a result, I am counting on you do your part at keeping this course environment safe and secure for all participants.

Enjoy!

Your Notes

Anny's Teaching

Let Us Have A Review

- Question 1 -
- Question 2 -
- Question 3 -
- Question 4 -
- Question 5 -

Your Notes

Anny's Teaching

Hypnosis For Medical Emergencies

Dr. Don Jacobs, Author, Psychologist and Emergency Medical Technician.

From this text on emergency care and transportation, from the Academy of Orthopedic Surgeons, briefly acknowledges a phenomenon that has been recognized in the healing arts for over 2000 years. In a medical crisis, a person's usual critical responsiveness to the environment may be altered so that information is subject to a literal translation that can either aggravate or support vital life systems

The communication of this information can thus affect physiological processes that are normally considered to be under the control of the autonomic or involuntary nervous system. Your words have the power to do untold harm, as the text states. They also have the power to create great benefit.

This program will go beyond the warning to merely avoid inappropriate conversation at the emergency scene. It will show you how to gain hypnotic rapport with a patient so that your words can tap that individual's enormous potential for coping. As a result, you can influence the course of vital functions.

Dr. Rachechas Jana is a Professional America of Physiology, an Internationally renowned researcher in neuro physiology in hypnosis. Dr. Jana states from his experience from clinical and experimental hypnosis in India during the past three decades:

After almost 30 years of research in neuro physiology and hypnosis, I found that any autonomic activity of the body and gland function can be altered by suitably uttered solutions in the hypnotic trance state.

Your Notes

Anny's Teaching

Such functions include: bleeding, immune responses, heart rate, blood pressure, respiratory functions, pain response, inflammation, alarm response, burn injury response, dermatitis and other nervous system functions.

David Cheek, M.D., is internationally recognized as an authority on medical hypnosis:

I am very happy to know that people who are dealing with emergencies - firefighters, police officers, are going to have a chance to use hypnosis because at a critical moment when people are either very frightened or unconscious, the primitive part of their mind is working for them, just as it does in hypnosis.

I was at a scene of an accident a few years ago where a woman was thrown through the top of her car and was lying underneath and her car was overturned on a little cliff. When I got to her, she was bleeding from an artery and her upper lip pumping. She was totally unconscious and not breathing even very regularly. I put my hand on her forehead and I said, "stop that bleeding, don't waste your blood." You got to give some sort of a command. That's the time when authoritative statements are worth doing. And it shows respect for the person's ability to stop their bleeding.

And I said, "the ambulance is on its way. Just relax and breathe evenly." And she stopped her bleeding. I went over to look at another woman that had been thrown out, who was in much better shape. I came back and there were some people sitting by her commenting on how dangerous it was for her to lie under that car. That there might be gasoline dripping on her, and she began to bleed again. And again, I pushed them away and told them to go look at the other person and I put my hand on her forehead again, just to attract attention and I said, "stop the bleeding, you did it the first time," and again she stopped. Very hard for people to understand to recognize that there is that much control of hemorrhage. It is a small artery, but the venous bleeding also can be stopped.

Your Notes

Anny's Teaching

People who are very frightened can be given a little description of what will be done next - that they'll go to the hospital and they will be taken care of. That they will be given treatment for whatever is the problem with them. Just to get them centered on something in the future, has a tremendous impact in the long range to use their own resources in recovering from injury. And I know as this use is extended as more credibility is given to those who are dealing with emergencies, there will be many lives saved, that are otherwise lost because of fear, because of hemorrhage, because of panic, unconscious panic and you are the ones that can do the most for the patient at that time.

The unconscious woman responded quickly to Dr. Cheek's confident directive to stop bleeding. Although a conscious person may or may not require more communicative preparation, it is seldom necessary for a first responder to induce hypnosis in an emergency victim in order for such suggestions to succeed. This is because emergency victims who are, or we believe they are, in a life-threatening condition, will automatically switch to an alternative level of mental perception. It makes them acutely responsive to images that they hold in their mind. This is what we call the hypnotic state of consciousness. Research shows that this transition may be a result of increased receptivity of certain image responsive chemicals such a neuropeptide.

These chemicals can be viewed as the brain's programmable software. Once triggered, they join with neurotransmitters in the brain, glands and immune system, to form a network of communication between the mind and the body. The sub non-critical acceptance of information initiated in the brain's primitive limbic system is probably a protective mechanism common to most animals.

During an emergency, it allows for quick and automatic compliance with the directions of a confident, trusted figure, such as the leader of a herd. In animals, external hypnotic directions come from body language, or other telepathic signals. In addition to these, man also responds to semantics or verbal communications. In the absence of such cues from the environment, the frightened individual depends on images that were

Your Notes

Anny's Teaching

associated with past experiences construed by the victim's subconscious to be related to the present problem.

Now if past images are inappropriate for the crisis at hand, which they often are, or if they are themselves negative or frightening, the survival mechanisms function below optimal capability. This is what happens to many emergency victims when the rescuers do not establish and utilize a positive hypnotic relationship with them. Since new, positive images can be reprogrammed at the emergency scene by the first responder who does do this, this is just a tremendous opportunity to positively influence a patient's survivability.

Lee Balance, M.D., is an emergency room physician and director of emergency services at Berkeley's Herrick Hospital:
A study of principles of hypnosis as outlined in this film can be extremely useful to first responders. The first contact that people make with the patient in distress can determine their outcome and their responsiveness to positive outcome at every level of care, from the field to the emergency room.

The person who understands the principles of hypnosis and is able to gain quick rapport to recognize states of spontaneous hypnosis can put themselves at a significant advantage in increasing the positive coping behavior of the patient and subsequent outcomes. I think that a trained paramedic who knows these principles can significantly augment my work in the emergency room.

The goal in this program is to present guidelines that will help you gain the patient's willingness to accept and act on your suggestions and directions, so as to achieve some of the results that have been described. It is important to remember while learning these emergency hypnosis skills, that they should be used only as an adjunct to standard medical treatment and not in lieu of it. To facilitate the learning process, these guidelines will be formulated according to the components represented by the acronym CREDIBLE:

Your Notes

Anny's Teaching

CREDIBLE

C = CONFIDENCE
R = RAPPORT
E = EXPECTATIONS
D = DIRECTIVES
I = IMAGES
B = BELIEVABLE
L = LITERAL
E = ENTHUSIASM

The four major components of hypnosis for medical emergencies include:

- The projection of **C**onfidence.
- Establishing and maintaining **R**apport with the patient.
- Developing positive **E**xpectations in the patient and,
- Giving proper **D**irectives and suggestions.

The acronym suffix describes the **D**irectives:

- They should invoke **I**mages.
- They should be relatively **B**elievable.
- It must be assumed they will be interpreted **L**iterally and,
- They should be given with appropriate **E**nthusiasm and conviction.

Confidence

The word "credible" itself is a reminder of an important aspect of hypnosis. Suggestions are more likely to be successful if there is a sense of credibility attached to them. Images must be believed in, if they are to be effective. This is why taboo death rituals work when they involve people who grow up in a culture that believes in them. Yet they would probably have little effect on you or I. So even though a victim in hypnosis is relatively uncritical of the suggestions per say, the more

Your Notes

Anny's Teaching

credibility given to the source of the suggestion, the more likely it is that they will be successful.

The first step toward assuring this sense of credibility is the projection of **C**onfidence. Before touching or speaking to the patient, you should take a moment to collect your thoughts and establish a course of action. Gaining confidence in using hypnosis may be a little challenging at first, especially amidst skeptical colleagues or other observers. However, as we begin to realize the potential of this kind of patient communication and you see how easy your words can help, you will soon be using hypnotic procedures without hesitation.

Captain Frank Neer, is an EMT in Orange County, California:

I have to admit I was rather skeptical when I first heard about the use of hypnosis in emergency situations, but after viewing the results obtained by trained personnel in the field, I came to be a little bit more than just barely amazed by results. Several incidents come to light when I think about the use of hypnosis in the field. One of the first ones that I think of right away was a little three year old girl that we had who was badly mauled by dogs. She had multiple lacerations and evulsions all over her body. She was hysterical and crying uncontrollably and starting to go into shock on our arrival. Within two minutes through the use of hypnosis, she was not only calmed down completely and helping in her own treatment, but the shock symptoms had begun to dissipate.

Another instance that comes to light when I start to think about some of the more dramatic uses of hypnosis; we had a 32 year old male who had suffered a 220 volt electrical shock. He was still breathing, although he had irregular and shallow respirations on our arrival and he still had a good heartbeat. He was undergoing seizure-like activity about once every minute and a half. Through the use again, of hypnosis, he was able to completely, or we were able to completely alleviate the seizure activity and to regulate his breathing back to a normal and deep respiratory manner.

Your Notes

Anny's Teaching

One of the last instances was probably one of the more dramatic for me. That was seeing an individual start and stop his own bleeding. We had a young man fall off his bicycle, landing on his head and causing a deep laceration of the scalp. As he did so, he got quite a bit of dirt and road debris into the wound and on our arrival, even though the bleeding had stopped, we were unable to tell the size of the actual wound itself and how bad it actually was because of the debris. On command, again a hypnotic command, he was made to start this bleeding process again, thereby cleaning out the wound and again a few moments later was told to stop the bleeding. It was nothing short of spectacular to see something like that actually occur in a simple situation. As I said, and I still maintain that even in the calls I go on today, I believe that hypnosis is a valuable tool for an effective treatment of the sick and injured.

Other first responders have had experiences and have drawn conclusions similar to those of Captain Neer. In 1975 the late M. Eric Wright, M.D., Ph. D., directed a six month long experiment comparing the patients attended to by a group of medics trained in hypnosis with the patients attended to by medics not trained in hypnosis. In a presentation before the American Society of Clinical Hypnotists, he described the results of the experiment, his disappointment that funds were not made available for further training of first responders and the fact that medics themselves became the ardent spokesmen for the use of hypnosis of emergency victims.

Dr. Wright was a world renowned psychiatrist who was widely acclaimed as a pioneer in the field of hypnosis. The following is a brief excerpt from his presentation just a few years before his death:

It seems absurd to find that such a relatively minor intervention, at least in the demonstration experienced that lasted six months, comparing the random patients that were picked up by the experimental crews, there were three crews; with the in-hospital care of those who were picked up by the non-trained crews, could make such a difference in first the number who were not dead on arrival, but who survived the trip, who were sustained and were able to be dealt with and who also had a quicker recovery rate. It is so absurdly simple that you really become terribly, at

Your Notes

Anny's Teaching

least I become terribly distressed that you can't budge administrative organizations to initiate this kind of practicing. There during the training, the ambulance drivers and those who are attendants. I think the drivers is not correct.

Those emergency personnel themselves became the proselytizers and we had difficulty keeping them from spoiling the experiment. You pardon my using this phrase and teaching others, "Hey really that guy really came through very nicely," and getting the feedback of them.

Until widespread training, teaching the skills introduced in this program is implemented, first responders who want to gain more confidence in using hypnosis should review and practice the strategies that will be presented. Reading the books listed at the end and taking courses offered by all qualifying institutions will also help.

For those whose confidence may be threatened by legal concerns, it should be noted that most states have no laws to charge from the use of hypnosis. And those few states that relegate it to the jurisdiction of physicians and dentists, medics simply need not label their communication strategies as being hypnosis, if they are worried about any repercussions.

In any case, it is important to remember that the emergency victim is already in the hypnotic state of consciousness and that you cannot harm anyone by offering positive, hopeful targets by detailing positive hopeful steps along the way.

In addition to studying and practicing the skills described in this program, another way to assure that you project confidence at the emergency scene is to practice self-hypnosis at home. A simple technique that can be used will also demonstrate how hypnosis affects the automatic physiological responses is by using a pendulum. Simply using a thread and a paper clip will do fine. But by holding the pendulum between your finger and thumb and allowing yourself to believe in the image of what would it look like if it began moving in a circle and not worrying about whether or not it happens, not trying too hard, but beginning to imagine it going around

Your Notes

Anny's Teaching

and round in a circle and while it is moving, seemingly automatically the ideomotor movements moving your pendulum, at that point you are entering into the hypnotic state of consciousness.
And in that state, a predetermined idea, or thought or goal in your mind, like confidence at the scene of an emergency should be visualized. And after several moments of visualizing that image, you can just allow yourself to return to a normal mode of consciousness.

1. <u>Sincerity</u>

Even with confidence you must establish a positive rapport with the patient before hypnotic directives are given. In many instances, rapport with a uniformed rescuer will be immediate. Such rapport can usually be maintained as long as you demonstrate sincerity, a proper balance of power and sufficient realism. Victims are sensitive to the sincerity or insincerity of those who are surrounding them. They will tend to focus their attention on the one who seems most sincere. That could be the rescuer or the stander-by who utters a damaging word.

2. <u>Balance of Power</u>

Although when an authoritative approach is sometimes appropriate, a bossy overbearing rescuer may lose rapport with the patient who requires more respect. The balance of power can be maintained if the rescuer a) acknowledges the patient's capability, b) says what he is going to do before he does it, and c) congratulates the patient on good responses.

Rapport

1. <u>Realism</u>

Comments that are obviously unrealistic can also break rapport. For example, saying that there is nothing to worry about to a person who just crashed his new car into someone's house will not give you much credibility. In many instances you may have to work a little to become

Your Notes

Anny's Teaching

the focus of the patient's hypnotic attention. The following strategies can be used to gain or regain positive rapport:

The quickest way to establish rapport is by simply asking for it. In the following dramatization, the victim agrees to do whatever the medic asks and immediately follows the suggestion to relax:

Lady: My arm! This really hurts, oh, oh!

Medic: Why, what happened here?

Lady: Oh I fell of the horse, oh, oh!

Medic: What hurts?

Lady: Oh my arm.

Medic: Okay, well I'm a medical technician with the Fire Department. The worst is over. I'm here to help. Would you do everything I say?

Lady: Yes.

Medic: Good. Why don't I go and check out your arm here, and why don't you concentrate on relaxing the rest of your body.

Lady: (heavy breathing)

Medic: That's good.

2. Feedback

Although it cannot hurt to attempt gaining a direct confidential rapport, indirect strategies often meet with more success, especially for the rest who is relatively inexperienced with hypnosis. With the feedback strategy, the patient comes to believe that the rescuer has a special knowledge about his or her feelings and thoughts and thus begins to focus attention on the rescuer's words. This can be accomplished by simply

Your Notes

Anny's Teaching

repeating things that are said by the victim or noticing things the victim is perceiving and then feeding back the information to them. In the following scene, a medic notices that the victim is becoming uncomfortable with the oxygen mask and uses this knowledge to gain rapport:

Medic: Rick, you might be concerned how that mask feels on your face. Most people are at first. What I would like you to do is just try and concentrate on breathing that cool comfortable oxygen and sending it to the parts of your body that need it. Good.

3. Joining In

Joining in is similar to feedback. With this approach, the rescuer joins in with the victim's feelings or actions to establish rapport and then gradually takes control of those feelings.

Dr. Helmut Rellinger, Ph.D., is a clinical psychologist in private practice in Berkeley, California, and an international speaker on hypnosis and related states:

Joining in is a useful hypnotic strategy when dealing with individuals who manifest extreme fear. For example, joining in with a desperate breathing rhythm of an asthmatic patient struggling for breath can help a rescuer gain that person's attention, and cooperation. First responders also frequently need to calm a hysterical patient or mostly our of control relative. Joining in strategies can be very helpful in such situations. Simply acknowledging the distraught person's feelings can have a noticeable calming effect. Thus instead of saying "It's okay, she's going to be fine. Just calm down", say "you are really scared, but we're going to take good care of him."

Acknowledging the person's emotional trauma can create instant rapport and make them much more compliant to subsequent instructions. Such an intervention can then be followed by a directive, which enlists the person's cooperation and involvement in the victim's care. An example of such a directive is, "I need you to help me take care of your husband.

Your Notes

Anny's Teaching

I need you to calm down, stand on that corner, and wait for the ambulance." Such directives should be meaningful to the person and partially distract them from the source of the emotional trauma.

Now this technique is especially useful in working with children. Children are much more likely to focus attention on an adult who understands how they are feeling, rather than how they should be feeling.

Lady: (having asthmatic attack)

Medic: I'm a medic with the Fire Department. I know how frightening it is not being able to breathe. Concentrate on my breathing and you will notice how easier it becomes to breathe. That's it, you're doing good.

Girl: (crying)

Medic: Hi Curra, boy, I'll bet that really hurts. Look at all that clean healthy blood. I bet that blood has cleaned that wound out pretty well now. I think you can go ahead and stop that bleeding. I have a pad here that you can put on there and hold on for me. Take your hand and put it over there. That's good.

Dr. Tom Stern, M.D., is a family physician and Director of the Berkeley Family Medical Group. He has lectured world wide on the use of hypnosis with children:

The first responder to a medical emergency involving a child has a tremendous opportunity, not only to make sure that the medical care is proper, but to give the child a quality of experience that will have influence later in life. If a child has psychological trauma in addition to the medical circumstances that are ongoing, it is quite common for them to develop deep-seated psychological disturbances around medical care and so it is particularly important to be dealing with it in a proper fashion. The natural coping abilities of children can be easily directed by the first responder to a medical emergency and according to techniques that are discussed in this tape by Dr. Jacobs, I believe that if every firefighter or emergency personnel were trained in the techniques described by Dr.

Your Notes

Anny's Teaching

Jacobs, that it would have an important influence on the medical outcome and the lives of a number of patients.

Medic: Curra, do you watch television? Do you watch Bugs Bunny on television? Well Curra, here is a little TV I have. Turn the TV on right there. Okay, and here's Curra and here's her dad and here's Bugs Bunny and they are all riding in the ambulance to the hospital. Doesn't it look like fun? Now if you want to see the TV again, just ask your dad and he will show it to you. All right. Okay.

4. <u>Diversion</u>

Another strategy for gaining rapport is to indirectly divert the patient's attention from his complaint. In the following scene, a secondary survey is used to do this. Each time a victim replies, temporary relief is afforded as focus is taken off the injury and rapport with the medic is enhanced.

Man: (moaning)

Medic: Rick, I am going to check the rest of your body to make sure things are okay. When I touch you on these parts, I want you to go ahead and lift this finger to let me know if it feels okay, all right? Let me touch right here. How does that feel? Okay, how about over here? Okay, good. And here, okay. How about over here? Good. And right here? Good.

There will be some times when it may not be possible for you to gain rapport with the victim. Usually this will happen with people who are on drugs, who are intoxicated or who are psychotic. However, it is sometimes possible to get such a person's attention and since the individuals are often in spontaneous hypnosis, you should continue to try gaining rapport until the patient is no longer in your care.

Once positive rapport is established, you may begin directing the patient towards the desired objectives. In hypnosis, each suggestion that is acted upon creates less opposition to successive ones. Therefore, when time permits, it is often best to begin with easier ones and work up to more

Your Notes

Anny's Teaching

dramatic ones. Each time the patient successfully follows a directive or suggestion, expectation is built up for implementing the next one.

Expectations

This brings us to the third letter of our acronym, standing for "expectation". The following strategies can be used to maneuver a victim to accepting beneficial suggestions. Once accomplished, expectations are then built for receiving subsequent directives.

Strategies For Building Expectation:

1. Contingency

In a contingency strategy, the desired suggestion is described as being contingent on the occurrence of something else that is going to happen for sure. In the following scene, the medic makes a suggestion for relaxation contingent upon the deflating of the blood pressure cuff. As the patient notices the cuff deflating, her subconscious automatically associates it with the contingent feeling of comfort. A variety of contingent actions can be used during patient treatment besides the one used for this demonstration:

Medic: Bea, now I am going to take your blood pressure. As the cuff deflates, notice how easier your breathing becomes. Good.

2. Double Bind

In a double bind strategy for building expectations, a patient is induced to follow a directive by offering him alternatives that all lead to the same results. In the following scene, the medic builds on the victim's own acceptance of comfort ability by setting up a double bind question.

Medic: Rick, I just want you to tell me if your arm is more comfortable here, across your belly, or if it is more comfortable here by your side? It is more comfortable across your belly, good. Notice that feeling of

Your Notes

Anny's Teaching

comfort coming up through your shoulder and going down through your torso and your arm.

3. Guided Imagery

Another strategy that is easily implemented and can result in increased expectations is to ask the patient to visualize a relatively easy image. Most patients will be surprised to see how easily they can be comforted by such an image or by how real it may seem. In the following scene the medic uses this strategy in conjunction with another that uses the patient's ideomotor movements.

4. Ideomotor Movements

Ideomotor movements of the fingers can be used to communicate with the victim and the automatic response of the finger gives the patient the expectation that special powers are at work.

Medic: Rick, I'll bet you can imagine there is some place you'd rather be right now. Why don' you go ahead and go there and let, in your mind's eye, and let me know when you get there by raising this finger. Good. Now I would like you to just relax there while we go ahead and get you ready for transport.

5. Elimination of Guilt and Anger

One way to progress with the giving of directives is to communicate with the patient in such a way to suggest that he not feel guilty or angry about the accident or illness. The mere elimination of guilt and anger will go a long way to make the patient feel better and he will tend to regard what you were going to say next with greater conviction and hope.

6. Belief in Hypnosis

Another way to build expectations is to directly ask the patient if they would like to use hypnosis to help them. If they say yes, just give your

Your Notes

Anny's Teaching

next suggestion by saying that it will occur when you count to three. If they say no, merely continue with another strategy.

It may take as little as ten seconds to project confidence, develop rapport and build expectations sufficiently for a hypnotic directive or suggestion to work. Remember that any autonomic nervous system function can be influenced in the patient who is in the hypnotic state of consciousness. Although it can generally be assumed that all frightened emergency victims are in a state, you will soon learn to recognize the signs of hypnosis.

Signs Of Hypnosis:

Some of the more obvious signs of hypnosis include tearing, eyelids fluttering, relaxed facial expression, slow speech, catalepsy and/or hyper suggestibility. A person in hypnosis may exhibit one or more of these characteristics. Of course, whether a patient is in hypnosis or not, you cannot hurt anything by giving hopeful suggestions that could enhance recovery.

Directives (Suggestions)

Although directives can relate to any autonomic nervous system function, they should always be structured with the following basic assumptions in mind:

1. Suggestions acted upon create less opposition to successive suggestions.

First, as we have already mentioned, any and every time a patient does something that is requested of him, the chances of success for later hypnotic suggestions is increased.

2. The Greater the concentrated effort, the less the subconscious response.

Your Notes

Anny's Teaching

The second assumption is that the more conscious and willful the effort, the less automatic the ability to respond. For example, the harder a patient tries to relax, the more difficult it will be.

3. What is expected tends to be realized.

The third assumption is what is expected tends to be realized. This is why it is helpful to build expectations before giving directives.

4. Imagination is more powerful than knowledge.

The fourth assumption is always keep in mind that imagination is more powerful than knowledge. Or to use Einstein's favorite quote "Imagination is everything." No matter what facts you might give to the patient, his or her imagined possibilities will create the response.

5. Every thought or image can cause a physical reaction.

And finally, every thought or image can cause a physical reaction. As illustrated by the pendulum effect involving ideomotor movements of the fingers.

One of the most dramatic demonstrations of the validity of these basic assumptions about hypnosis relates to hypnotic intervention with burn injuries. Few injuries are as traumatic as severe burns. Of the 300,000 injured by fire every year, nearly 50,000 lie in hospitals for a period ranging from two months to two years. And many must return again and again for painful reconstructive surgery. Furthermore, relatively few hospitals provide specialized burn care.

In those that do, more and more physicians are recognizing the value of hypnosis in treatment. Although suggestions for vasodilatation to the burn sites, significantly augment healing when given several hours post-burn. The most dramatic influence occurred when suggestions for vaso construction to the burn site are given within one hour post-burn. This is especially useful for firefighters to know because they are likely to be the first to reach the victim or an injured fellow firefighter.

Your Notes

Anny's Teaching

If the burn victim was given the hypnotic suggestion to imagine a feeling of coolness and comfort within the first hour of the burn, before normal and physiological and psychological responses take effect, a significant reduction in burn injury and enhancement of healing can occur. The burning, pain and swelling are due to the nervous system's inflammatory response and these can be remarkably controlled.

According to Dr. Larry Moore, a medical hypnotherapist who works with burn patients, the first responder who reaches the victim within this time frame of one hour, and gives hypnotic suggestions of being cool and comfortable, might well save the life of that individual.

I am very pleased to have the opportunity to make this brief presentation to you because I am convinced that firefighters, paramedics – those who are first on the scene, the first to respond to burn victims, have a tremendous potential not only to influence their immediate comfort, which we all know about, but also to affect their healing and even the depth of their wounds.

We have had on occasion, patients brought into the burn centre that I have seen within the first hour of post-burn and by immediately giving them essentially hypnotic icing of the burn wound, we find that by the next day, they are less deeply burned than we thought on intake. We have even seen in a couple of patients who were at intake, said to have third degree burns, and the following day the surgeon in charge of the burn will say, "well, it looks like it is only a deep second degree burn," which has a tremendous difference.

This was a patient who would have had to be grafted over 60% of his body, instead he had a second degree burn, which could be healed without resorting to grafting and without the common scarring and problems.
So you see that you have the opportunity right on the spot to make a tremendous difference, as I said, not only in comfort, but in wound healing, in wound depth and I don't think it is far fetched at all to say on the morbidity and mortality. You may save a person's life by this.

Your Notes

Anny's Teaching

Jerold Kaplan, M.D., is director of the acclaimed burn centre at Alpha Beta's Hospital in Berkeley, California:

First responder understands the basic principle of hypnosis. They have a significant effect both initially and from the long-term outcome of a burn victim. The first responder who gets there within minutes of the injury can lessen the effect of the burn injury by giving suggestions to the patients of cool and comfortable. This is an internal form of cooling, similar to the external form of cooling that might be utilized by the application of ice water or other cold liquids. The techniques are simple, effective and may be used by anyone at any time.

In addition with cooling, will also give the patient pain relief from his injury so that you are adding two aspects. Decreasing the possibility of progression of the injury, as well as making the patient more comfortable during the initial transport to appropriate definitive medical care. The techniques have been utilized for some time, are well documented and effectively decrease burn injury.

I utilized this one time on my son, who had come back from bad sun exposure during skiing, and we talked about cool and comfortable on his face. The next morning when he woke up, his face had no effect and normally this might just be that he was not going to have a burn anyway. Except that his ears, which we had not mentioned and which he did not internalize as part of his face, were bright red. A simple, effective rapid technique that can and should be used by any first alert responder.

Dabney Ewin, M.D., is a physician with the Occupational Health Centre in New Orleans, Louisiana. Dr. Ewin is internationally recognized as one of the foremost researchers on the use of hypnosis with burn victims. The following photos graphically illustrate the effectiveness of Dr. Ewin's hypnotic treatment of patients.

This patient of Dr. Ewin's was given hypnotic suggestions for being cool and comfortable immediately after he was burned. Anatomically in a black person, the pigment layer is in the basement membrane of the skin, so this is a deep second degree burn of the face. This picture shows the

Your Notes

Anny's Teaching

patient on the fourth day after injury. Note that there is no swelling, not even of the eyelids, nor did the patient use any medications besides aspirin.

This photo was taken six weeks after the injury. According to Dr. Ewin, burns of this sort usually require at least four months of disability before return to work instead of six weeks, which is common with burns that Dr. Ewin treats with hypnosis.

Another of Dr. Ewin's patients is burned on the arm by an acetylene torch when the hose broke. The jet blast from the torch was sufficient to vaporize the patient's shirt and charcoal the outer layers of his skin. Dr. Ewin hypnotized the man within one hour of the event and using cool towels, he gave suggestions to keep it cool and comfortable until it was healed.

This picture shows the first dressing at 21 hours post-burn. Dr. Ewin does not scrub the injured areas and simply applies the dressing over the charcoal. Note that at 21 hours, there is no edema or swelling about the burn and there is even wrinkling of the skin distal to the burn.
At 8 days, you can see the outer layers of charcoaled skin are peeling off and there is healthy skin beneath. At 12 days, there is no scar tissue and no permanent burn scar.

Your Notes

Anny's Teaching

Images – Rules for Giving Directives

In addition to the basic assumptions regarding hypnotic directives, the following guidelines will ensure that each suggestion or directive meets the four basic objectives represented by the suffix of our acronym. So doing will help guarantee that each directive will elicit the desired physiological and psychological response.

1. Be Descriptive:

The first set of guidelines will help cause the directive to produce an image in the patient's mind. The first rule is to be descriptive. Don't merely say, for example, "your heart is beginning to work fine." Instead

say, "your heart muscle is becoming stronger. The muscle fibers are now working together in an effort to pump blood into your arteries."

2. Be Simple:

While you want to be descriptive, you must be careful not to be complex. Avoid long, technical words. Speak to each victim as if you were talking to a bright ten year old. For example, it is better to say "working together in a team effort," than "working together in a coordinated effort."

3. Use Emotional, Exciting Words:

The third way to help ensure an image is formed with your suggestions is to use emotional and exciting words. Listen to the excitement and emotion in this suggestion:

You have a wonderful temperature control in your body that is now ready to start working as you begin to imagine being sprayed by a cool mist of clear water. You might even notice how it feels to have an equally cool, comfortable breeze bring your temperature back to where you feel comfortable.

Your Notes

Anny's Teaching

4. Use Native Language When Possible:

When possible, working with a bilingual person, it is easier using an image when you speak to them in their first language.

The second group of rules will help make the record believable enough to be accepted by the victim.

Believable

1. Use Progressive Form of the Present Tense:

The first rule is to use the progressive form of the present tense whenever giving your suggestions. This gives the patient time to work up to the idea. For example, saying "notice how much easier your breathing is becoming" is preferable to "your breathing is much easier now."

2. Be Accurate:

Accuracy will help make suggestions believable also. For example, don't say "everything will be all right," instead say , "the worst is over." Similarly, don't tell a patient that all the discomfort will go away if it won't. Instead, use a scale of one to a hundred, with one being the most comfortable and one hundred being the least comfortable and move them down to an acceptable level.

3. Make Suggestions Relative to the Patient:

Make suggestions relative to the patient, not to the environment or others. Be sure that your suggestion relates specifically to the patient's responses and not to the responses of others. Don't ask, for example, to imagine the sun is getting cooler when its not. Instead, have them imagine a more appropriate response to the heat of the sun, or don't tell them that the attendants at the emergency room will all be friendly. Instead have them concentrate on having them react to abrupt treatment with a positive attitude.

Your Notes

Anny's Teaching

Literal

The third factor to remember when giving suggestions is that your words will be interpreted literally by the victim.

1. <u>Avoid phrases that have more than one meaning:</u>

By avoiding phrases that have more than one meaning, you minimize the chances of causing inappropriate response to your suggestions. Putting someone to sleep may mean something different to an anesthesiologist than it does to the individual who just put their German Shepherd.

2. <u>Affirm Activity, Not Ability:</u>

Remember to make your suggestions relative to what the patient is beginning to do and not to what they are able to do. If you tell someone that they have the ability to breathe normally, they may accept this suggestion literally and they indeed believe they have the ability, but they will not act on it since you did not tell them to do so.

3. <u>Be positive, Avoid Negative Phrases and Words:</u>

Because of the patient's literal perception of phrases, it is important to only use positive words. For example, if you say, "you are beginning to feel less pain", the negative word "pain" reinforces the fact that the patient has pain. By saying, "you are now beginning to feel more comfortable", this problem is avoided. Similarly, don't use a negative phrase like, "you are not going to die." The patient's image producing mind will not pick up words like "not" and will focus on the more visual words like "die". Instead of saying, "you are not going to die", say, "you are continuing to live and going to continue living."

Your Notes

Anny's Teaching

Enthusiasm

The last component of our acronym is a reminder to use the right amount of enthusiasm in giving your suggestions or directives. Too much enthusiasm may worry the victim. Too little may negate the impact of your words. If your directives are given with sincerity and confidence and are following all the rules we have discussed and they still don't seem to be working, increase your projection of enthusiasm and see what happens.

Help the victim to see the situation as a challenge rather than a problem, as challenges are more likely to be dealt with enthusiastically.

Once you have completed your medical treatment and manage the victim with appropriate hypnotic suggestion, it is probable that the patient will be transported into a hospital emergency room by someone other than yourself. A hypnotic directive aimed at giving the patient an independent opportunity to keep his life systems functioning optimally should be given, especially if the next EMS tier is unfamiliar with hypnosis procedures. This can be done with a general directive for wellbeing, coupled with what is called a trigger. The trigger is a simple ritual that the individual can perform to be reintroduced to hypnotic suggestion on his own in times of need:

Medic: Okay Ray, the ambulance will be here in a few minutes. Things are being made ready for you at the hospital. Your body is already beginning to heal itself. All your body systems are doing exactly what they need to be doing to make you heal rapidly and whenever you feel the need to, you can touch just your finger and thumb together and you will notice that cool and comfortable feeling come flooding back into your arm and leg. Go ahead and touch your finger and thumb together now. Good.

Your Notes

Anny's Teaching

If the next tier of EMS support is familiar with hypnosis, the first responder can easily transfer the victim's rapport with himself to the new rescuers. This is done by simply introducing the conscious or unconscious victim to the rescuers, telling him that he will be in capable hands, and then telling the rescuers what hypnotic capabilities the victim has managed to achieve.

Hopefully some day all EMS providers will come to realize that the most powerful healing force of all is the human mind.

The use of hypnosis in emergency situations present both an opportunity and a challenge to all emergency personnel.
The opportunity is to develop patient communication at a level that may enhance creative and possibly life saving physiological responses.
The challenge is to break through the barrier of bias preconception and mind sets that deter objective evaluation.

Dr Thomas Elmmendorf, MD.

===

Your Notes

Anny's Teaching

Questions About Hypnosis For Medical Emergencies

- Question 1 -

- Question 2 -

- Question 3 -

- Question 4 -

- Question 5 -

Your Notes

Anny's Teaching

Fright, Stress And Words

During fright, a particular image held in the mind will bring about a particular effect

Attributed to Hermes + - 8,000 BC

During periods of great stress, words that seem immaterial or are uttered in jest might become fixed in the patient's mind and cause untold harm.

American Academy of Orthopedic Surgeons, 1987 AD

Your Notes

Anny's Teaching

Body – Cell Regression

Just as the Soul has a past, the body has a past too, and it is found in the body's cells.

Something that truly runs in the family (like haemophiliacs) is a disease passed from either the sperm or the egg and can be found with body-cell regression.

Let us compare the Soul, our no-physical self to the driver of our car, our physical body. When we go back into past experiences of the Soul, we go to past lives.

Each of the parts of a car have a history: the quality and where the material comes from, the scratches, the accidents, and so forth. You can "read it" that by learning psychometry. The car is our physical body. The physical body has a history too, as it's inherited genes, the DNA. The process of passing an illness and a curse happens by a highly charged emotion.

A physical condition is then impregnated by a highly charged emotion frozen in the sperm or the egg and passed at the time of conception, and by going back to the cause, we can clear it.

Remember, it has been proven that the DNA responds to the way we think, just like a car starts to ride a certain way by the way we drive it. A car who was only driven in a city by a overly cautious person will be very sluggish on the highway.

Once we reach the cause, the situation and the emotion that froze itself in either the egg or the sperm, we can repair it.

I learned this from Yvette Eastman, an exceptional and highly advanced Kinesiologist who shared with me her experiences with her clients as she learned more and more how to apply kinesiology, a fascinated as well as very structured method of healing.

Anny Slegten

Your Notes

Anny's Teaching

Psychometry

Divination of facts concerning an object or its owner through contact with or proximity to the object.
From: *Webster's' New Collegiate Dictionary*

Scientists Prove DNA Can Be Reprogrammed By Words And Frequencies

By Grazyna Fosar and Franz Bludorf

THE HUMAN DNA IS A BIOLOGICAL INTERNET and superior in many aspects to the artificial one. Russian scientific research directly or indirectly explains phenomena such as clairvoyance, intuition, spontaneous and remote acts of healing, self healing, affirmation techniques, unusual light/auras around people (namely spiritual masters), mind's influence on weather patterns and much more. In addition, there is evidence for a whole new type of medicine in which DNA can be influenced and reprogrammed by words and frequencies WITHOUT cutting out and replacing single genes.

Only 10% of our DNA is being used for building proteins. It is this subset of DNA that is of interest to western researchers and is being examined and categorized. The other 90% are considered "junk DNA." The Russian researchers, however, convinced that nature was not dumb, joined linguists and geneticists in a venture to explore those 90% of "junk DNA."

Their results, findings and conclusions are simply revolutionary!

According to them, our DNA is not only responsible for the construction of our body but also serves as data storage and in communication. The Russian linguists found that the genetic code, especially in the apparently useless 90%, follows the same rules as all our human languages.

Your Notes

Anny's Teaching

To this end they compared the rules of syntax (the way in which words are put together to form phrases and sentences), semantics (the study of meaning in language forms) and the basic rules of grammar. They found that the alkaline of our DNA follow a regular grammar and do have set rules just like our languages. So human languages did not appear coincidentally but are a reflection of our inherent DNA.

The Russian biophysicist and molecular biologist Pjotr Garjajev and his colleagues also explored the vibrational behaviour of the DNA. [For the sake of brevity I will give only a summary here. For further exploration please refer to the appendix at the end of this article.]

The bottom line was: "Living chromosomes function just like solitonic/holographic computers using the endogenous DNA laser radiation." This means that they managed for example to modulate certain frequency patterns onto a laser ray and with it influenced the DNA frequency and thus the genetic information itself. Since the basic structure of DNA-alkaline pairs and of language (as explained earlier) are of the same structure, no DNA decoding is necessary.

One can simply use words and sentences of the human language! This, too, was experimentally proven! Living DNA substance (in living tissue, not in vitro) will always react to language-modulated laser rays and even to radio waves, if the proper frequencies are being used.

This finally and scientifically explains why affirmations, autogenous training, hypnosis and the like can have such strong effects on humans and their bodies. It is entirely normal and natural for our DNA to react to language. While western researchers cut single genes from the DNA strands and insert them elsewhere, the Russians enthusiastically worked on devices that can influence the cellular metabolism through suitable modulated radio and light frequencies and thus repair genetic defects.

Garjajev's research group succeeded in proving that with this method chromosomes damaged by x-rays for example can be repaired. They even captured information patterns of a particular DNA and transmitted it onto

Your Notes

Anny's Teaching

another, thus reprogramming cells to another genome. ?So they successfully transformed, for example, frog embryos to salamander embryos simply by transmitting the DNA information patterns! This way the entire information was transmitted without any of the side effects or disharmonies encountered when cutting out and re-introducing single genes from the DNA.

This represents an unbelievable, world-transforming revolution and sensation! All this by simply applying vibration and language instead of the archaic cutting-out procedure! This experiment points to the immense power of wave genetics, which obviously has a greater influence on the formation of organisms than the biochemical processes of alkaline sequences.

Esoteric and spiritual teachers have known for ages that our body is programmable by language, words and thought. This has now been scientifically proven and explained.

Of course the frequency has to be correct. And this is why not everybody is equally successful or can do it with always the same strength. The individual person must work on the inner processes and maturity in order to establish a conscious communication with the DNA. The Russian researchers work on a method that is not dependent on these factors but will ALWAYS work, provided one uses the correct frequency.

But the higher developed an individual's consciousness is, the less need is there for any type of device! One can achieve these results by oneself, and science will finally stop to laugh at such ideas and will confirm and explain the results. And it doesn't end there…

The Russian scientists also found out that our DNA can cause disturbing patterns in the vacuum, thus producing magnetized wormholes! Wormholes are the microscopic equivalents of the so-called Einstein-Rosen bridges in the vicinity of black holes (left by burned-out stars).

These are tunnel connections between entirely different areas in the universe through which information can be transmitted outside of space

Your Notes

Anny's Teaching

and time. The DNA attracts these bits of information and passes them on to our consciousness. This process of hyper communication is most effective in a state of relaxation. Stress, worries or a hyperactive intellect prevent successful hyper communication or the information will be totally distorted and useless.

In nature, hyper communication has been successfully applied for millions of years. The organized flow of life in insect states proves this dramatically. Modern man knows it only on a much more subtle level as "intuition." But we, too, can regain full use of it. An example from Nature: When a queen ant is spatially separated from her colony, building still continues fervently and according to plan.

If the queen is killed, however, all work in the colony stops. No ant knows what to do. Apparently the queen sends the "building plans" also from far away via the group consciousness of her subjects. She can be as far away as she wants, as long as she is alive. In man hyper communication is most often encountered when one suddenly gains access to information that is outside one's knowledge base.

Such hyper communication is then experienced as inspiration or intuition. The Italian composer Giuseppe Tartini for instance dreamt one night that a devil sat at his bedside playing the violin. The next morning Tartini was able to note down the piece exactly from memory, he called it the *Devil's Trill Sonata.*

For years, a 42-year old male nurse dreamt of a situation in which he was hooked up to a kind of knowledge CD-ROM. Verifiable knowledge from all imaginable fields was then transmitted to him that he was able to recall in the morning.

There was such a flood of information that it seemed a whole encyclopaedia was transmitted at night. The majority of facts were outside his personal knowledge base and reached technical details about which he knew absolutely nothing.

Your Notes

Anny's Teaching

When hyper communication occurs, one can observe in the DNA as well as in the human being special phenomena.

The Russian scientists irradiated DNA samples with laser light. On screen a typical wave pattern was formed. When they removed the DNA sample, the wave pattern did not disappear, it remained.

Many control experiments showed that the pattern still came from the removed sample, whose energy field apparently remained by itself. This effect is now called phantom DNA effect.

It is surmised that energy from outside of space and time still flows through the activated wormholes after the DNA was removed. The side effect encountered most often in hyper communication also in human beings are inexplicable electromagnetic fields in the vicinity of the persons concerned.

Electronic devices like CD players and the like can be irritated and cease to function for hours. When the electromagnetic field slowly dissipates, the devices function normally again. Many healers and psychics know this effect from their work. The better the atmosphere and the energy, the more frustrating it is that the recording device stops functioning and recording exactly at that moment. And repeated switching on and off after the session does not restore function yet, but next morning all is back to normal. Perhaps this is reassuring to read for many, as it has nothing to do with them being technically inept, it means they are good at hyper communication.

In their book *"Vernetzte Intelligenz"* (Networked Intelligence), Grazyna Gosar and Franz Bludorf explain these connections precisely and clearly. The authors also quote sources presuming that in earlier times humanity had been, just like the animals, very strongly connected to the group consciousness and acted as a group.

To develop and experience individuality we humans however had to forget hyper communication almost completely. Now that we are fairly stable in our individual consciousness, we can create a new form of group

Your Notes

Anny's Teaching

consciousness, namely one, in which we attain access to all information via our DNA without being forced or remotely controlled about what to do with that information.

We now know that just as on the internet our DNA can feed its proper data into the network, can call up data from the network and can establish contact with other participants in the network. Remote healing, telepathy or "remote sensing" about the state of relatives etc.. can thus be explained.

Some animals know also from afar when their owners plan to return home. That can be freshly interpreted and explained via the concepts of group consciousness and hyper communication. Any collective consciousness cannot be sensibly used over any period of time without a distinctive individuality. Otherwise, we would revert to a primitive herd instinct that is easily manipulated.

Hyper communication in the new millennium means something quite different: **Researchers think that if humans with full individuality would regain group consciousness, they would have a god-like power to create, alter and shape things on Earth! AND humanity is collectively moving toward such a group consciousness of the new kind**. Fifty percent of today's children will be problem children as soon as the go to school. The system lumps everyone together and demands adjustment. But the individuality of today's children is so strong that that they refuse this adjustment and giving up their idiosyncrasies in the most diverse ways.

At the same time more and more clairvoyant children are born [see the book *"China's Indigo Children"* by Paul Dong or the chapter about Indigos in my book *"Nutze die taeglichen Wunder"*(Make Use of the Daily Wonders)]. Something in those children is striving more and more towards the group consciousness of the new kind, and it will no longer be suppressed.

As a rule, weather for example is rather difficult to influence by a single individual. But it may be influenced by a group consciousness (nothing

Your Notes

Anny's Teaching

new to some tribes doing it in their rain dances). Weather is strongly influenced by Earth resonance frequencies, the so-called Schumann frequencies. But those same frequencies are also produced in our brains, and when many people synchronize their thinking or individuals (spiritual masters, for instance) focus their thoughts in a laser-like fashion, then it is scientifically speaking not at all surprising if they can thus influence weather.

Researchers in group consciousness have formulated the theory of Type I civilizations. A humanity that developed a group consciousness of the new kind would have neither environmental problems nor scarcity of energy. For if it were to use its mental power as a unified civilization, it would have control of the energies of its home planet as a natural consequence. And that includes all natural catastrophes!!!

A theoretical Type II civilization would even be able to control all energies of their home galaxy. In my book "Nutze die taeglichen Wunder," I have described an example of this: **Whenever a great many people focus their attention or consciousness on something similar like Christmas time, football world championship or the funeral of Lady Diana in England then certain random number generators in computers start to deliver ordered numbers instead of the random ones. An ordered group consciousness creates order in its whole surroundings!**

When a great number of people get together very closely, potentials of violence also dissolve. It looks as if here, too, a kind of humanitarian consciousness of all humanity is created. (The Global Consciousness Project)

To come back to the DNA: It apparently is also an organic superconductor that can work at normal body temperature. Artificial superconductors require extremely low temperatures of between 200 and 140°C to function. As one recently learned, all superconductors are able to store light and thus information. This is a further explanation of how the DNA can store information.

Your Notes

Anny's Teaching

There is another phenomenon linked to DNA and wormholes. Normally, these super small wormholes are highly unstable and are maintained only for the tiniest fractions of a second. Under certain conditions stable wormholes can organize themselves which then form distinctive vacuum domains in which for example gravity can transform into electricity.

Vacuum domains are self-radiant balls of ionized gas that contain considerable amounts of energy. There are regions in Russia where such radiant balls appear very often. Following the ensuing confusion, the Russians started massive research programs leading finally to some of the discoveries mentions above.

Many people know vacuum domains as shiny balls in the sky. The attentive look at them in wonder and ask themselves, what they could be. I thought once: "Hello up there. If you happen to be a UFO, fly in a triangle." And suddenly, the light balls moved in a triangle. Or they shot across the sky like ice hockey pucks.

They accelerated from zero to crazy speeds while sliding gently across the sky. One is left gawking and I have, as many others, too, thought them to be UFOs. Friendly ones, apparently, as they flew in triangles just to please me.

Now the Russians found in the regions, where vacuum domains appear often that sometimes fly as balls of light from the ground upwards into the sky, that these balls can be guided by thought. One has found out since that vacuum domains emit waves of low frequency as they are also produced in our brains.

And because of this similarity of waves they are able to react to our thoughts. To run excitedly into one that is on ground level might not be such a great idea, because those balls of light can contain immense energies and are able to mutate our genes. They can, they don't necessarily have to, one has to say.

For many spiritual teachers also produce such visible balls or columns of light in deep meditation or during energy work which trigger decidedly

Your Notes

Anny's Teaching

pleasant feelings and do not cause any harm. Apparently this is also dependent on some inner order and on the quality and provenance of the vacuum domain. There are some spiritual teachers (the young Englishman Ananda, for example) with whom nothing is seen at first, but when one tries to take a photograph while they sit and speak or meditate in hyper communication, one gets only a picture of a white cloud on a chair.

In some Earth healing projects such light effects also appear on photographs. Simply put, these phenomena have to do with gravity and anti-gravity forces that are also exactly described in the book and with ever more stable wormholes and hyper communication and thus with energies from outside our time and space structure.

Earlier generations that got in contact with such hyper communication experiences and visible vacuum domains were convinced that an angel had appeared before them. And we cannot be too sure to what forms of consciousness we can get access when using hyper communication. Not having scientific proof for their actual existence (people having had such experiences do NOT all suffer from hallucinations) does not mean that there is no metaphysical background to it. We have simply made another giant step towards understanding our reality.

Official science also knows of gravity anomalies on Earth (that contribute to the formation of vacuum domains), but only of ones of below one percent. But recently gravity anomalies have been found of between three and four percent.

One of these places is Rocca di Papa, south of Rome (exact location in the book "Vernetzte Intelligenz" plus several others). Round objects of all kinds, from balls to full buses, roll uphill. But the stretch in Rocca di Papa is rather short, and defying logic sceptics still flee to the theory of optical illusion (which it cannot be due to several features of the location). All information is taken from the book *"Vernetzte Intelligenz"* von Grazyna Fosar und Franz Bludorf, ISBN 3930243237, summarized and commented by Baerbel. The book is unfortunately only available in German so far. You can reach the authors here: www.fosar-bludorf.com
Transmitted by Vitae Bergman[www.ryze.com/view.php?who=vitaeb]

Your Notes

Anny's Teaching

Anchoring

As I explained, during HYP 203, anchoring can be done in many ways for may reasons.

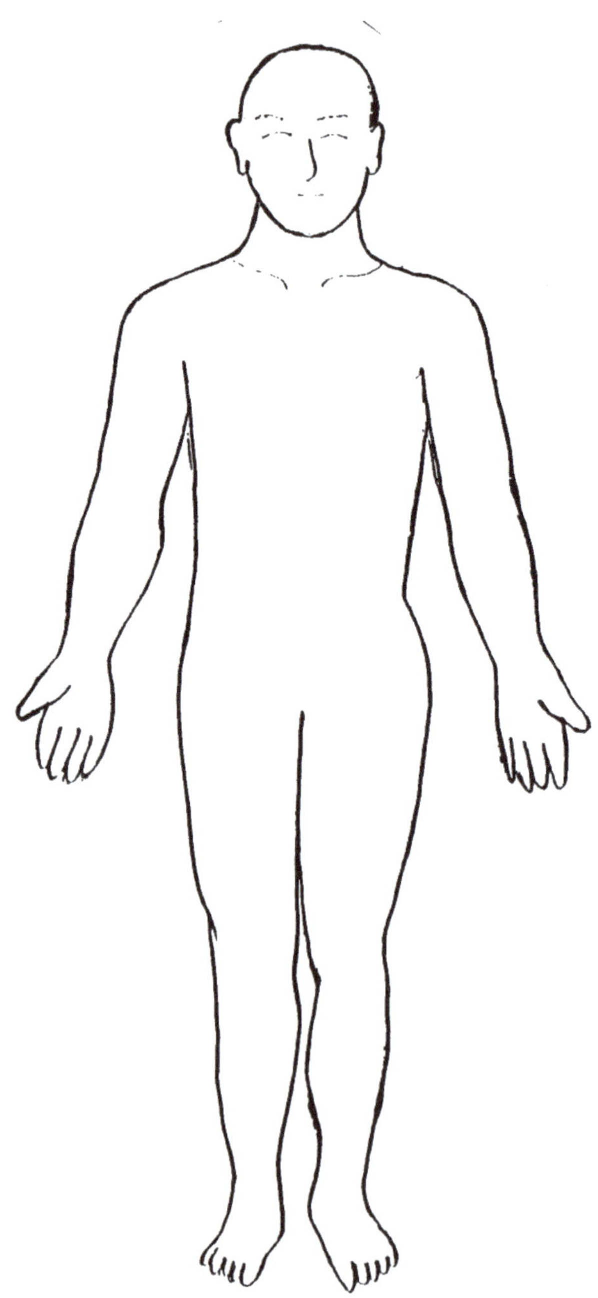

Your Notes

Anny's Teaching

Emotional Stress Release – An Emotional Lift

A Review

At the end of a session, very effective in putting the client back together for clarity of thoughts so the event/issue becomes a story

Please note: sometimes, the Emotional Stress Release becomes a complete session when a client comes to retrieve the memory of a past event or when a client comes to your office in a high level of stress and confusion.

At the end of the session, lightly hold the frontal eminence with one hand and the Primary Visual Areas with the other hand.

- Ask the client to review the session and all the insights gained through the session.

- Ask the client to go to the cause of what was affecting him/her and review how it affected him/her from then all the way to now.

- When finished, ask the client to rewind the movie of time from now all the way to the beginning at twice the speed it took to review it.

- Repeat several times

- Ask the person to review the whole thing and to stop to what she/he perceives is the crucial point in the series of events., and to stop it at the top of ther head.

Your Notes

Anny's Teaching

- As the client stops at the significant event, instruct him/her to review the issue simultaneously from where she/he stopped back to the beginning and from where s/he stopped all the way to now at the speed you will move your hands from the frontal/occipital holding to the top of the head and back to the frontal/occipital holding.

- Have the client do this complete exercise until you feel a continuous pulse. Take your time and allow your client to go through this at their own pace. The results are worth it.

When appropriated, put the problem in a container and have it sent to the sun, etc.

Variations

When used to have a clear information, each time the client goes back, I ask my client to go "further back in time", and review everything from then on to now.

Note: Sometimes, once in a trance, the client draws a blank and replies "nothing" to any suggestions. Do, then, the complete exercise, asking the client to go to the beginning of the "nothing" and review the "nothing" from the beginning all the way back to now, etc., have the "nothing's" residues put in the container, and so forth. The results are the same!

Your Notes

Anny's Teaching

Circuit Retaining Mode

This is a method I learned taking courses in Touch For Health in the mid 1980's. As I was observing the method, I realized that, since we can connect physically, taking on a person's energy, doing all the muscle corrections and then release the corrected energy back to its rightful owner, we certainly could do that by connecting psychically, and thus the method to do surrogate hypnotherapy sessions was developed.

First, drink water to insure a good "connection".

What follows is part of the class material on the subject received during these Touch For Health workshops.

We are able to put information into a "retaining mode" in the biocomputer by putting the information "in circuit". This is like having an endless tape message, on a telephone answering machine, feeding the message we want into the computer's awareness all the time.

Any testing we do, or correction we make, when something is in circuit is now made in relation to the information "on hold" in this retaining mode.

The "circuit retaining mode" (or "Pause Lock" as it is sometimes called) consists of moving the feet 18 inches or more apart at the time we are activating whatever information we want held "in circuit". As we move the feet apart a huge amount of sensory information from both femur heads converges on the brain. Other information arriving with it is blended with it and held until the feet are moved together again. (The brain defocuses off the femoral head information and focuses on the material that arrived with it, giving the effect of the "endless tape". This is like a radio receiving the carrier wave and the sound signal blended as one impulse. The radio tuned to amplify only the signal, not the carrier wave.)

Your Notes

Anny's Teaching

Either the testor or the testee can hold the circuit as their energy fields become blended by touch during balancing. (The testor therefore can act as a "surrogate retaining mode" so long as touch is maintained).

Source: Webster's New Collegiate Dictionary:

Femur: 1- the proximal (closest) bone of the hind or lower limb – called also *thighbone.*

Practice Of Circuit Retaining Mode

Understanding the use and effectiveness of emotional stress relieve.

Read the emotional level of client, get into their energy field and record what you 'read'

Then do the emotional stress release

1. Drink some water (Both your client and yourself) to make a good "connection"
2. Have your client sit in an upright chair and think of something they are emotional about.
   - Explain the purpose of this technique is for "it" to become a story.
3. Ask client to think about "it"
   - Put your legs together and touch the client as they are contemplating "it" and go in the "circuit retaining mode"

Your Notes

Anny's Teaching

4. Check the feelings in your own body, feelings belonging to your client.

- Write it down and cancel the "circuit retaining mode".

5. Do the Emotional Stress Release technique on "it"

6. At the end, say to client …"when your subconscious mind has made the decision as to when the issue will end – whether now, an hour from now, later today, tomorrow, next week, whenever – then you will be able to open your eyes, feeling much better in many ways"…

7. Put yourself "in circuit" again as you ask your client to contemplate "it" and touch the client while they are doing so.

8. Check the feelings and compare the results to your notes. Cancel the circuit.

9. Holding their head in the Emotional Stress Release mode, instruct your client to contemplate "it" and go to the beginning, the middle and then to the end of "it", wherever it is.

10. Ask client for a verbal feedback on how they feel about "it" If required, put yourself "in circuit" to check things out and then cancel the 'Circuit".

11. If still a feeling, holding their head in the Emotional Stress Release mode, have client go back to the beginning of "it, the middle and then the end of "it".

When necessary, do the complete emotional stress release again, having held to the issue or simply pretended they did it, not wanting to do the work.

Your Notes

Anny's Teaching

Practice – In A Few Words

1. Ask your client to contemplate the situation that annoys them.
2. In the Retain Circuit Mode, read the client's energy and write it down.
3. Perform the complete Emotional Stress Release.
4. Putting yourself back into the Circuit Retaining Mode, ask the client to contemplate the situation that annoys them as you read the client's energy. If still the same, re-do the Emotional Stress Release.
5. Reads the client's energy again. When fine, when appropriated, use the Container.
6. Wrap it up.

Your Notes

Anny's Teaching

Post Accident Trauma Release

Release of what is contained in the aura: Body Trauma from Current and Past-Life Traumas

A one day course given by Paul Hansen, Ph.D. at the Association of Past Life Research and Therapies conference given in San Francisco, CA in the Summer of 1990.

Introduction to Accident Trauma Release (ATR)
by Dr Paul Hansen.

We sometimes see patients who show the residual effects of an accident or other body trauma that occurred earlier in their lives.
Medical feedback shows that the body has – or should have – healed, but for some reason it has not released the memory of the event.
Such patients often have chronic pain and "know" something is wrong, but doctors cannot find the problem. Out of my effort to understand and treat this phenomena, the technique of post traumatic release (ATR) was born. After three years of learning and experiencing, I have begun to share ATR. Feedback indicates that others are also having rewarding results.

Three years ago I was working with a woman I'll call Nancy, who had been in continuous pain since an auto accident a year and a half earlier. She had been driving at night in a snowstorm. Her windshield had become clogged with snow, and she got out to scrape it. While she was doing so, a truck hit her car from behind, causing her car to throw her end-over-end through the air until she landed on her head in a snow bank. She was unconscious for several hours and afterward had little recall of the accident.

Under hypnosis, she went back over the accident several times, moment by moment until she recalled it all, including exactly how her body landed. Various points of her body seemed to hold some of the "shock energy".

Your Notes

Anny's Teaching

The body can be thought of as a gelatinous mass held up by the skeleton. When a shock impacts the mass, the energy goes to the other side and then ricochets back and forth until it gradually comes to a still point. Whenever the kinetic energy changes directions, some seems to be collected and held in the tissues. In Nancy's case, the energy rippled again and again through her body in a surprising way. Her whole body seemed to readjust as certain points were released.
Explain this to the client prior to starting the session

To understand why this treatment was successful, I began to research the field but have found only the beginning of a theoretical base.

Marcel Vogel, a researcher at IBM who developed the magnetic tapes and disks, concludes from his research the body cells store memory in a way similar to the magnetic media used in computers. The body stores information in other areas as well as in the brain cells. Broken bones or damaged tissue can develop a parasitic energy imbalance like a psychic or energetic cancer,

The mind has no mechanism for accessing why the injury took place and cannot release the damage.

Dr Herbert Spiegel, a psychiatrist who used hypnosis to treat men who had war-related psychiatric trauma, concluded that the men's symptoms protected them from the memory of the horror of the events. The therapeutic goal was to separate the memory from the horror, so that the event could be remembered without the initial emotional reaction.

ATR can be extended to past-life trauma, especially those that are carried over into pain in this life. For instance, a man who had pain in a rib all his life experienced – though past-life regression – a life as a gold miner, during which life he was hit in the rib by a log when a dam broke. Release through the ATR process caused the pain to cease. Often some current-life trigger assists in the initial recall of the past-life trauma.

\

Your Notes

Anny's Teaching

ATR adds something significant to simple recall of the trauma. The special-temporal precision that the patient can bring to finding the focus or locus of the trapped energy is surprising. Focus on the exact point where the energy is trapped brings a tremor, while a quarter-inch deviation brings no response.

A phenomenon known in physics as piezoelectric shows that when a piece of metal is bent or an attempt is made to bend a piece of living bone, its electrical balance is changed – the compressed side becoming negative and the stretched side positive. Perhaps this ionic change could influence the “memory” of a bone. My hypothesis is that, on a tissue level, there is a change in the molecular rhythm or pattern of the cell salts, which is replicated when the cell divides, becoming coded into the DNA. The therapeutic release reprograms the cells in the area of the injury to reestablish a “normal” pattern.

The Thalmic Neuron Theory of pain mediation postulates that when a massive pain signal comes from a nerve or group of nerves through the thalamus, it over-excites that nerve body and leaves it permanently vibrating, continuing to send pain signals to the brains – even if the body part has been amputated. When the nerve is re-stimulated, as by acupuncture, the neuron of the nerve is jiggled out of its firing pattern and is allowed to return to normal homeostasis.

In doing research on Therapeutic Touch at the University of Colorado Medical Center, we have used a device called SQUID (Super Quantum Interference Device) in which the sensor is kept in liquid helium so that the superconductor can pick up the electromagnetic changes in the environment around the body. This device, called a Magnetoencephalograph, can pick up extremely minute electromagnetic emanations, making possible an excellent magnetocardiogram of the aura. The ATR may be related to these energy fields or systems.

Your Notes

Anny's Teaching

We are still in an exploratory phase in understanding how this new process works to facilitate healing in the body, but total theoretical understanding is not necessary to use the process in clinical practice.

Paul A. Hansen, Ph.D., Th.D., has a psychotherapy practice in Denver and has been doing past-life therapy for many years. In 1990, Paul Hansen was on the Association of Past Life Research and Therapies Board and was Chairman of the Training Committee.

Your Notes

Anny's Teaching

Steps Of The ATR Process

NOTE:

Client and Facilitator to drink water to facilitate a good connection

1 - Milton Erickson's Typical Induction

A - Abdominal breathing, taking twice as long on the exhale as on the inhale.

B - Use a metaphoric image of turning off switches in the body to induce relaxation in adjacent muscles. Ask the patient to imagine the switch, then turn it off and indicate by "OK" when he has done so. Suggest that the body part will be relaxed, heavy and warm.

The sequence is:

- right foot, right knee, right hip,
- left foot, left knee, left hip,
- right hand, elbow and shoulder
- left hand, elbow and shoulder
- throat area, neck
- shoulders, upper back
- forehead and face,
- top of the head
- base of the spine

Your Notes

Anny's Teaching

Suggest that as the entire lower part of the body goes into a deeper relaxation, the patient's awareness will become crystal clear.

- Top of the spine at the base of the skull

Suggesting that the upper part of the body is even more relaxed, heavy and warm.

C - Repeat the abdominal breathing, taking twice as long on the exhale as on the inhale.

2 - Deepening

A - Invite the patient to imagine a vertical scale from 1 to 100 and indicate what number approximates his level for relaxation, one being the deepest.

B - Say that as you count from ten to one the patient will go deeper and deeper. Count slowly, interspersing count with suggestions for relaxation.

C - Ask again for the patient's location on the vertical scale.

3 - Clarifying the Accident or Trauma

A - Ask the patient to go back to the accident or trauma. Say "You will count from one to five and that at five he will be able to describe all events clearly". Ask for a description of physical sensations and any movement of the body.

(I find it much more effective and easier on my client when I hold the client's head as in the EMOTIONAL STRESS RELEASE technique – Anny)

Ask for all details. Have the client repeat the complete story three times.

B - Go back through the event in ultra-slow-motion. Go to a fraction of a moment before impact.

Your Notes

Anny's Teaching

Say that when you count to three the patient will be there. Then move to the moment of impact. Ask you client often "How do you feel?" to keep the client in an hypnotic trance.

4 - Trauma Release

A - Say, "I will place my fingertip where you have described the impact to be (Name this)
Help me to find the exact spot".

B - Say, "We will release all pain and trauma from this place in your body. I will count to three. Notice where the energy goes, as it may ricochet around the body.

One, two, three, release! ". ***ON THE EXHALE***
(As you count, touch the traumatized spot (***very gently***)
"Help me know where it where it went"

(When necessary, help client by practicing the circuit retaining mode.)

C - Follow the energy to the next spot and release in the same manner. Continue until all the energy spots have been released.
(It is my experience that when the body starts to release all the trauma and "wakes up to life", the client will start to tremble – streaming - as it is called. Anny)

At that point, have the client observe the complete event from outside of their body,
asking the client how they left their physical body and then ask them where is their energy body now in relation to their physical body.

This is what is called Soul Retrieval.
And then proceed at directing the client in integrating both bodies. Suggest it is like putting a wetsuit on, wiggling their toes, pulling the wetsuit up, etc.

Your Notes

Anny's Teaching

Once completed, encourage the client to let go of the sound of how it feels for the energy body to be integrated again in the physical body. Sometime, the sound of the agony of the soul is something you will vividly remember.

Instruct the patient to retain the changes and suggest that the body will continue its healing process. Continue these suggestions as you count the patient back to regular consciousness.

Your Notes

Anny's Teaching

Questions about Soul Retrieval

- Question 1 -

- Question 2 -

- Question 3 -

- Question 4 -

- Question 5 -

Your Notes

Anny's Teaching

Soul Retrieval

Our thoughts are non physical and so is the mind that sends impulses to our physical brain.

Since our thoughts are affecting our life, it is understandable that we are in fact much more energy beings than physical beings.

We live two lives, and the physical life is accommodating the energy life who is usually two years ahead of our physical self. Yes, there is a parallel life. My clients taught me that physical death usually occurs two years after a severe trauma or a decision to die.

For the longest time, I thought that we were 25 % physical and 75% pure energy. To my observation, I came to the realisation that we are in fact 5% physical and 95 % pure energy, and when these two parts are not synchronised, physical and/or mental dysfunctions are occurring.

When not wanting to face life, been totally in the energy space while we have a physical body feels great. We do not feel our physical self when we are out of it. However, while being a "space cadet" makes one oblivious to what is going on around them, life goes on and during moments of lucidity one resents what is going on. Street drugs may create that condition too.

Have you notice? A child runs, falls and then after a moment of silence starts to cry. Their energy body propelled out of the physical body kept running, and then, realising there is something missing, returns into the body and then feels the pain.

Being partially out of the body is another story. There is then a physical uneasiness, and to bring a person back to full synchronization is what is commonly known Soul Retrieval.

Your Notes

Anny's Teaching

When practicing physiological stress release, ask your client to view the event from an out of body vantage point and without realising it, your client in a deep trance will explain how they left their physical body and then how they are back into it… and how the two bodies are attached now.

A client had a heart attack while driving a tractor in a field. A nurse driving by noticed it, stopped her car off the highway, jumped over the field fence and proceeded to pump his chest to get him back to life. When I saw him, his life was in disarray.

During the session he discovered only his physical and energy hearts were in sync, the balance of his two selves were totally out.

Sometimes I ask my clients to lift themselves up and then come back into their physical body, aligning their two selves properly. There are many variances. The importance is to get them back in full alignment. To facilitate this, I ask my client to consider their energy body as a wet suit they are putting on. The results are surprising: bones getting back in place, the feelings back in a limb, just to mention a few.

This has also something to do with a Near Death Experience.

Your Notes

Anny's Teaching

Consciousness Is Everywhere

The Missing Link

In all the research one does for an article such as this, there comes a realization that "out there" there is a missing link.

For example, to believe that consciousness arises from matter entirely misses the link between matter, and its original source.

By that measure, matter came into being spontaneously – from where? And how?

In addition, at least some researchers in the field of neuroscience are still wondering when and how consciousness first arises in a newborn child.

What might they think of this excerpt from an article by Dr. Mercola?

''Plants communicate with other plants – even with plants of other species through a complex underground network that includes:

1. The plants, rhizosphere (root ball)
2. Aerial emissions (volatile gasses emitted by the plants)
3. Mycelial networks in the soil

"These three systems work together forming a 'plant internet' of sorts where information about each plant's status is constantly exchanged."

Your Notes

Anny's Teaching

Consciousness Is Everywhere: It Is All In The Mind

A Harvard University study published in 2008 found the first compelling evidence that the Relaxation Response (RR) – the physiological response to meditation, yoga, tai chi, Qi Gong or repetitive prayer – affects our genes.

"Now we have solid scientific proof of the positive genetic effects of meditation in that it affects genes that positively influence cell metabolism and the response to oxidative stress."

It's in our own mind that "higher thought frequencies" can be initiated.

Your Notes

Anny's Teaching

Mindfulness

To my understanding, it is a technique now known as Mindfulness.

This is an article my friend Yvette Eastman had sent me, as she explained I most likely know this and sent it to me anyway!

Al Sears, MD
11903 Southern Blvd., Ste. 208
Royal Palm Beach, FL 33411

March 09, 2009

Dear Yvette,

The University of Iowa took brain scans on pain suffers and found results that were remarkable.1 They could actually *see* the parts of the brain that experience pain shutting down. How did they do it? They used a technique that will surprise you.

The lead author of the study, an anesthesiologist, said he thinks this technique is approximately 65% - 70% effective against pain.

A panel of experts at the National Institutes of Health said the same thing. They found that this technique can fight pain of all kinds. I am not just talking about headaches. The research revealed that it can work for painful conditions from chronic illness to irritable bowel syndrome.

Even mainstream media is on board. *The Wall Street Journal* said, “Numerous scientific studies have emerged in recent years showing that the [technique] can exert a real and powerful effect on the body.”

I have some good news: You can teach yourself this technique with the right guidance, in the comfort of your own home. It is medical hypnosis.

Your Notes

Anny's Teaching

It is a scientifically proven way you can beat pain – without the dangerous side effects of pain medications.

Here is just one example you can try at home. It is based on an ancient form of breathing meditation from India called *vipassana.*

1. Get yourself into a comfortable position. It can be sitting in your favorite chair, on the sofa, even lying down in bed.

2. Make sure your environment is as quiet as possible. Turn off the TV or radio, have the kids go play outside—whatever it takes to create a peaceful, still atmosphere.

3. Close your eyes and begin gently focusing your attention on your breathing. Breathe naturally, without trying to control it. Do this for about 5 minutes, so that your mind settles down a bit and your body feels relaxed.

4. Gently let your attention rest on the source of your physical pain, keeping your eyes closed. With each breath, focus gentle awareness on the place where the pain happens.

5. Now imagine breathing "into" that place. Allow your attention to rest in the area of the pain and breathe in with gentle awareness. You can even place your hand over the area.

6. Imagine your pain responding to your breathing by "opening up" and slowly disappearing. Do this for 5 to 10 minutes, however long is most comfortable for you.

7. Complete your meditation by bringing your awareness back to your breath for a minute or so and opening your eyes.

This is an effective way to change your experience of pain over time. You are teaching your body to "relax" with the pain. This keeps it to a minimum. I know it sounds funny, but you will see real results if you stick to it.

Your Notes

Anny's Teaching

I learned this technique from a medical hypnosis expert named Dr. Maggie Phillips. She has been training doctors all over the world for years on how to use your mind to reduce and control pain. She is someone I have come to trust.

Dr. Phillips put together a four-CD course, ***Hypnosis: The Pain Solution***, which I offer folks here at my Wellness Center. My patients tell me it really works. One 47-year-old man I will call Jose struggled for years with habit-forming pain medications. He said:

"Since adding Maggie Phillip's guided hypnosis to my daily regimen, I have improved dramatically. I stopped using prescription drugs everyday. The amount I take now is almost down to zero."
To Your Good Health,

Al Sears MD

Schulz-Stübner et al. "Clinical hypnosis modulates functional magnetic resonance imaging signal intensities and pain perception in a thermal stimulation paradigm." 2004. *Regional Anesthesia and Pain Medicine*. 29(6):549-556.

"Integration of Behavioral and Relaxation Approaches into the Treatment of Chronic Pain and Insomnia." NIH Technology Assessment Statement. October 16-18, 1995. 1-34.

Michael Waldholz. "Altered States: Hypnosis Goes Mainstream: Major Hospitals Use Trances for Fractures, Cancer and Burns, Speeding Surgery Recoveries." *Wall Street Journal*. October 3, 2007.

Your Notes

Anny's Teaching

Variation On A Theme

Reiki Energy Exercise

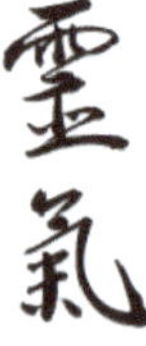

Reiki Undo

Reiki (energy) exercise

Workshop Hand-Out

The breathing technique Reiki Undo was devised by Mrs Koyama, the sixth president of the Usui Reiki Ryoho Gakkai. The Japanese word Undo means exercise. Sit or stand in the Gassho position and pray for the Reiki energy to come through you. Say to yourself: Reiki Undo begin. If you are practicing with a partner, touch his/her shoulders from behind and allow the body to move, whichever way it wants to move. Breathe in deeply and let go as much as you can when you are breathing out. After a few deep breaths your body will probably start to move.

If the movement does not come through you easily, be patient and don't create anything. Keep doing this exercise for at least three months on a daily basis.

***Anny Slegten's notes* :**

This is an exercise to be done once a day.
Energy radiates from our entire body.
This is an exercise to let the energy move our body so it can regulate itself to good health.

Take a few deep breaths and let the body move.

Your Notes

Anny's Teaching

It can take some time before the body starts to move, therefore simply « jump start » the process. In the beginning you will have to « jump start » several times before getting into the mode.

To jump start:

Thumbs in, arms extended forward, breathe in.

Breathe out as you tense your body, bring the elbows back to your body and totally let go as you go into the « mode ».

By letting the energy move the body, the energy moves the blocks and the body starts to discharge the toxins and functions properly.

When alone, follow your body needs 10 to 40 minutes.

In a group, the energy usually slows down after 10 minutes.

When « coming back », quietly look at the body from the inside.

There is a similar technique in Indonesia called «TOUYOU».

Note :

When I observed the demonstration I found it looked very much like when Ramtha enters J.C. Knight's body and aligns his energy to the body he entered.

Your Notes

Anny's Teaching

The Laser Fox, The Laser Hoe

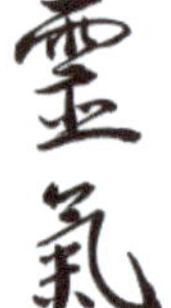

Fox Technique or
Kangaroo Technique

The Laser Fox. The Laser Hoe.

No Workshop Hand-outs given

Anny Slegten's notes **(« Table work »)**

There is some similarity with the « Tripod » technique learned from Reiki Master/Teacher Trish Dennison and the « Ultrasound » technique in Healing Touch.

This is also taught by a branch of the Reiki Alliance.

Left hand : all fingers touching the left thumb.

Right hand : the two central fingers touching the right thumb.

We were instructed to work on a partner laying on a table, look at the person holding the left hand turned up all fingers touching the left thumb with the intent of connecting and receiving Universal Energy. Close our eyes and imagine we have X-Ray vision of the person and let the laser (right hand) just hover above the person where the energy guides us.

Please understand we all have our personal way to experience the « X-Ray vision ». For me, I see thick black lines on the body where my « laser » is directed.

During this exercise, I saw a thick black line along the bottom of the rib cage. My hand got stuck above Margo's navel and a sharp pain made my

Your Notes

Anny's Teaching

hand jump. I then gently drew « it » out, and that was it. Standing there, eyes closed, the X-Ray vision went blank. I opened my eyes, looked at Margo and put both hands on her lower arm.

Later, Margo explained her stomach burped and the discomfort vanished (an indigestion from too much coffee at breakfast that morning).
Margo also thanked me for putting both hands on her arm ! Nobody had touched her since she left home to take several courses three weeks prior to this one and it comforted her to be touched on the arm.

Your Notes

Anny's Teaching

Tibetan Psychic Surgery

It is preferable to have the person you will be working on lay down in front of you.

In our mind, you have a shelve in front of you where you will find spare parts and place a disposable container close to you to either your left or your right side.

First ask the person where the issue is according to them.
As you are getting ready to do the healing, look at the person laying in front of you, take a deep breath, close your eyes and go into n hypnotic trance.

Scan the body, hovering your hand over the issue. You will have a distinct feeling of where the issue is located.

Remember to trust your hand since sometimes the issue is not where the person thinks it is.

Your yes still closed, remove that part and place it in the disposable container. Then, reach for a new spare part on the shelf and insert it to where you have removed the part. If it does not fit, place the new part back on the shelf and replace it with another part. Do this until you get the right one.

The new part must fit.
Finish the process with anything you feel needs to be

Your Notes

Anny's Teaching

Now Is Your Turn To Ask Me Questions!

- Question 1 -

- Question 2 -

- Question 3 -

- Question 4 -

- Question 5 -

Your Notes

Anny's Teaching

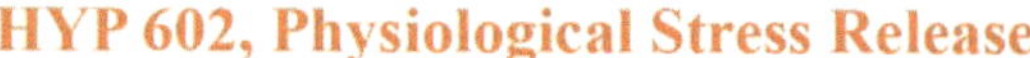

Dedication

Remember the poster I gave you at the end of HYP 202?

It was a poem found in Henry Ford's desk drawer in his wife's handwriting.

Well, here it is:

> ***Bite off more than you can chew and chew it.***
>
> ***Dare to take on more than you can do and do it.***
>
> ***Hitch your wagon to the stars,***
>
> ***Keep your seat,***
>
> ***And there you are!***

Well, it is what kept me going when I put all the hypnosis class material in book form now available on Amazon.

Considering my computer skills, I took on more than I could chew – that is for sure! Without the incredible help I got from four people, I am sure I would not even look at such a mammoth project.

It all started with Boomer who, while in training, one day showed up in class with the incredible, beautiful *Hypnotism Training Institute of Alberta, Canada* Coat of Arms.

With enthusiasm, he then proceeded to put all the *HYP 101 Hypnotism, an Introduction* class material in book form.

Colin then made it compatible to be printed by Amazon.

Marietta, who was at the time basking in the sun on a beach somewhere during a bitter winter here in Alberta, Canada designed the HYP 101 book cover on her very smart Laptop. Thankfully, she had taken it along, for "Just in case." Following this, she designed the Kimberlite Publishing House logo.

After publishing HYP 101 on Amazon, it took Colin three years to persuade me to do the same with each of the next class materials for the rest of the courses.

Because of the way the course material could now be presented in class, the quality of the in class discussions was incredible!

As usual, I needed to see the end result in my mind.

And then, various events happened – including the Covid-19 virus. It was the right time to give the school a rejuvenated two shots, just like me getting vaccinated with two jabs in the arm for total protection.

Pat, my Webmaster went along and rejuvenated my websites, as well as being excellent at 'cleaning' pictures – These pictures became a highlight of the front covers of the six Class Companions.

Colin, having already published six books on Amazon, was doing the book layouts, as well as having suggested what to put on the front and the back of the book covers.

Having gone to her office to choose the colours, Marietta created and designed the templates as well as the striking book covers to project what I wanted to convey.

Colin had an incredible patience with me – coming to the office, correcting my work as I was watching him. I watched to learn to outsmart that electronic machine who, in my view, is as temperamental as a woman.

A soon as you figure out how to handle the computer, an UPDATE appears – and you have to figure it all out again! Right?

Typing this class material often got me in a pleasant hypnotic trance, and as I am reading what I typed, the spellcheck was in a hypnotic trance too!

In addition to have come to the office from 8:00 am to 11:00 am well over 20 times, I was also calling Colin on the telephone many times, asking how to get out of a situation that, according to the computer, I got myself into.

It got taxing for him, and Colin gave me a hypnosis session as a HYP 202 class demonstration – fixing my computer "thing."

And it worked well – much to his surprise and delight.

Result: The six HTI Class Companions published on Amazon in seven months.

Yes, this was really teamwork.

As the present saying goes: "We are all in this together"… that we like it or not.

From the bottom of my hearth – I thank each and every one of them to have helped me.

Anny Slegten

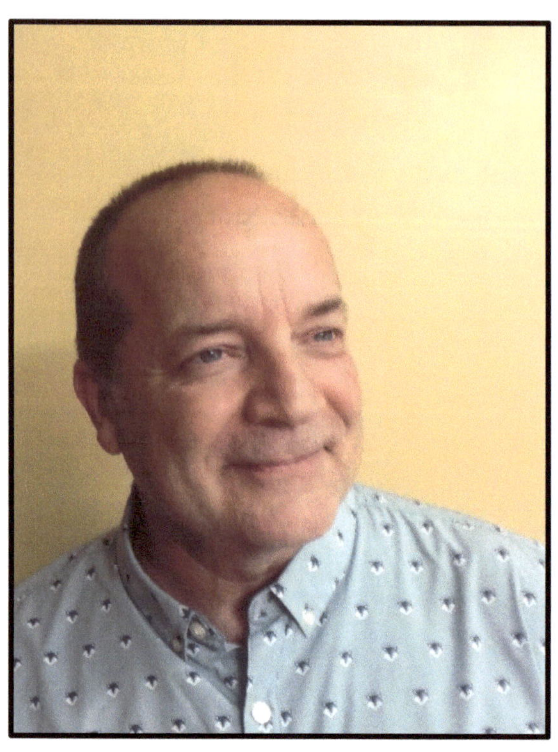

Boomer Stralak

Very creative and master of all trades.

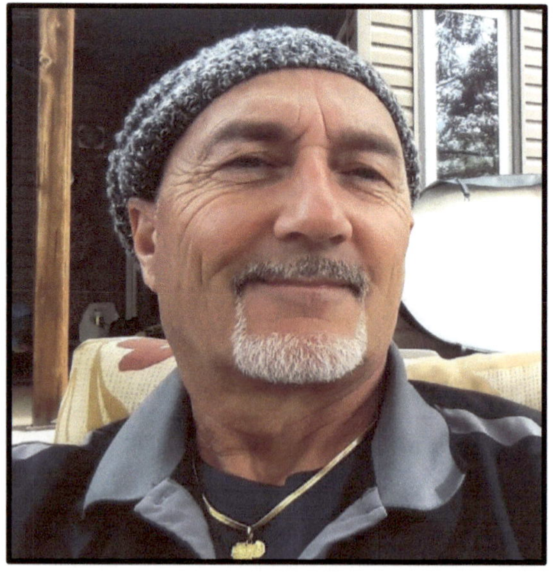

Patrick Perka

Next Phase Multimedia
Graphic & Web Design
Multimedia Project Management
Edmonton, Alberta, Canada

www.NextPhaseMultimedia.com

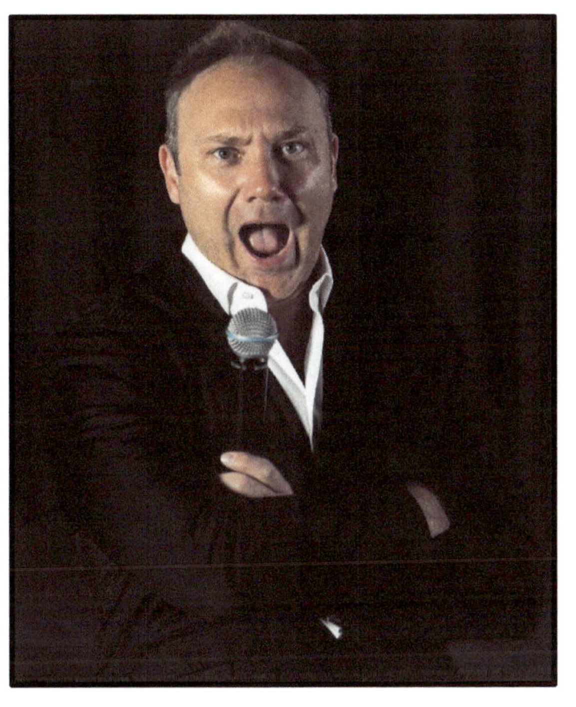

Colin Christopher

Colin a keynote speaker, presents clean and funny corporate stage hypnosis comedy shows.

Colin also teaches online marketing and selling courses as well as teaching stage hypnosis in person.

www.colinontv.com
www.colinchristopher.com

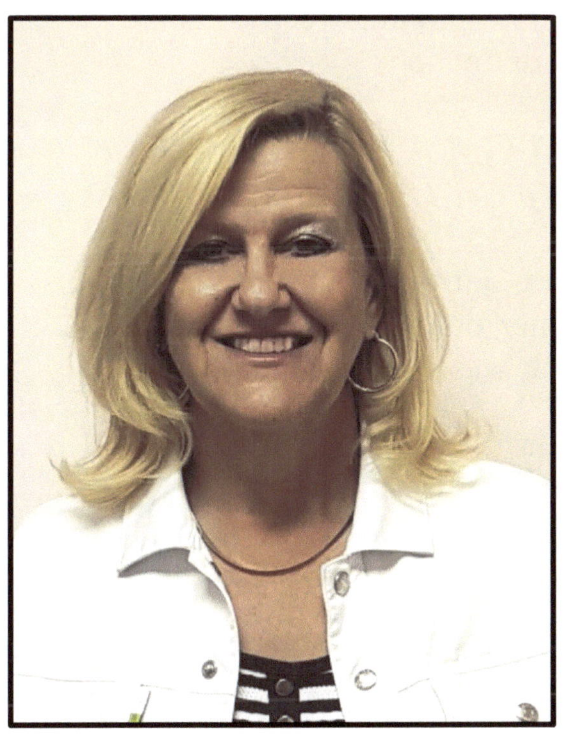

Marietta Miller

Logo and brand development
Print and Marketing Materials
Advertising and Direct Mail Campaigns
Publishing

www.execugraphx.com

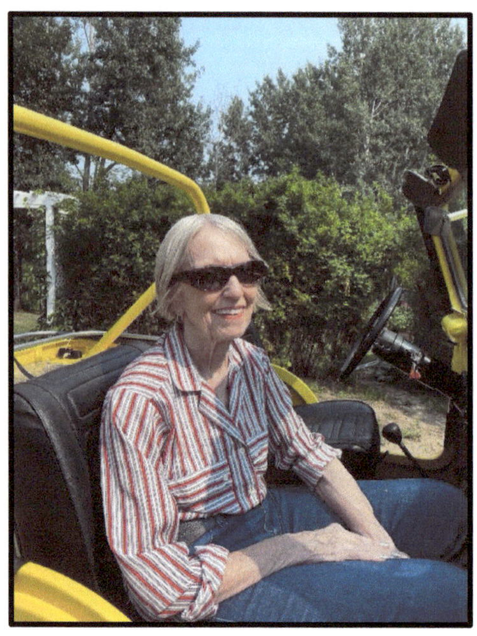

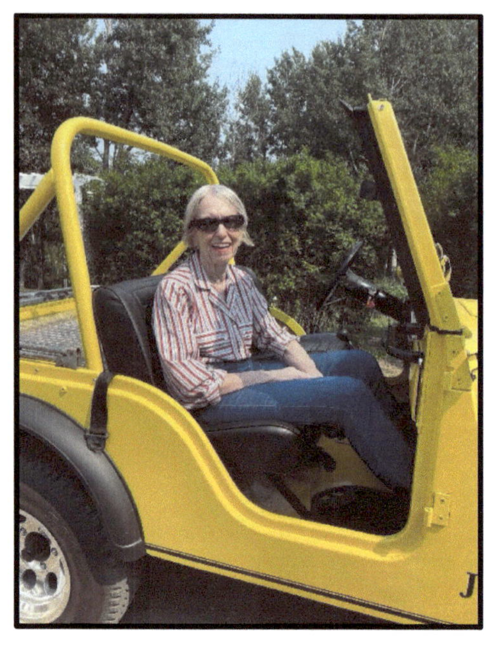

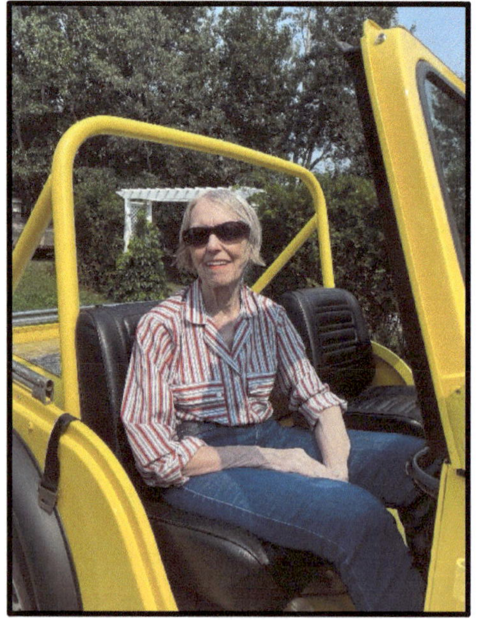

This is the 1977 Willis Jeep I am writing about in my book

And Then I Got A Blue Carpet
How To Get Things fast

Her engine was purring with pleasure when taking her out for a ride on my 85th birthday. It was a beautiful day, no tarp needed.

Please note: There were no safety belt when we bought the Jeep brand new, only a "chicken bar" on the dashboard for the passenger to hold on to for safety.

Afterword

Congratulations! As you completed 319 hours of in-person class training and all your many hours reviewing and completing the homework I gave you – I really admire you.

You have now earned the designation of Certified Clinical Hypnotherapist.

I really wonder if you acknowledge who we are as human beings.

We are powerful people. We have the ability to manipulate our environment to our liking – many times not foreseeing the package deal we ended up with.

After our body released our Soul, we enter the planning stage and review the physical journey we just left. It is our Soul that writes the script of our next physical life.

We do this, wanting to shake off something that sits heavily on our conscience. With this information, we then decide the physical body our soul we will be wearing.

It is much like deciding on what coat we wear when we go out into the weather.

Earth is not a restful place. We all need the courage to be honest with ourselves and at peace with it. Our Soul wanted us to resolve and evaluate our physical life experience and accomplishments on this Earth.

I know this is work – spelled W.O.R.K.

The problem is: While in the planning stage, writing the script of our next physical experience – we do not ask for "the pleasure of" resolving whatever we want to resolve. Because of this, we many times end up living a nightmare.

Yes, we are the one's who designed it that way. As uneasy as it is to admit it: There are no victims. We are all volunteers.

Having studied hypnosis in all its forms and applications – you now have the tools to help those who ask for help on hand. This allows their Soul to succeed at putting closure on what weighs heavily on their conscious.

In an emergency situation when the oxygen masks are coming down, a flight attendant explains perfectly: "Put the mask on you first, and then help someone who needs help."

Therefore, in earnest – have the courage to work on yourself. Ask for help when needed.

Let us face it:

We have the freedom to choose to resolve whatever has to be resolved in present time. Or, we keep our head in the sand – then having to come back (reincarnate) to accomplish what our Soul had decided to resolve and dissolve this time around.

It is our very own decision, our choice.

Each and everyone of us volunteered the life we are experiencing at present time.

With freedom comes responsibility.

Acknowledging our responsibility and doing something about whatever needs to be done, results at experiencing an incredible and sought out peace of mind.

The challenge?

Forgiving ourselves for having gotten off track.

You know I care. This is the reason I am reminding you of it all.

And from the bottom of my heart, thank you for reading me.

Anny Slegten,
Instructor,
Hypnotism Training Institute of Alberta, Canada

...

Online Store, Contact, And More…

You may contact Anny by visiting any of her websites and scroll down the home page to the contact information.

http://www.annyslegten.com
Anny's private website and online store.

http://www.success-and-more.com
To find the description of the many services offered, and more.

http://www.htialberta.com
The Hypnotism Training Institute of Alberta including descriptions of hypnosis and hypnotherapy courses given.

http://www.reiki-canada.com
About the Reiki Training Centre of Canada.

http://www.slegtenianhypnosis.com
Although open to anyone interested in this fascinating hypnosis modality, this website information is for graduates of the Hypnotism Training Institute of Alberta.

http://www.connectwithanny.com
This is the best place to keep up to date with Anny – including seeing all her latest books and how to order them on Amazon.

Other Books By Anny Slegten…

REIKI PURE AND SIMPLE

Volume I: The Sacred Rites

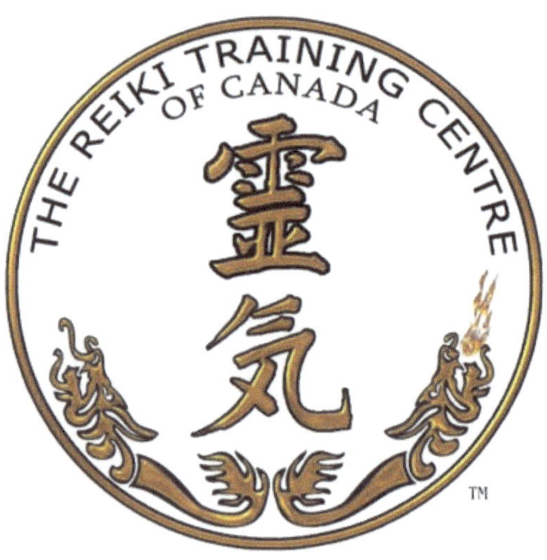

Anny J. Slegten

Reiki Training Centre of Canada
Class Material
http://www.reiki-canada.com

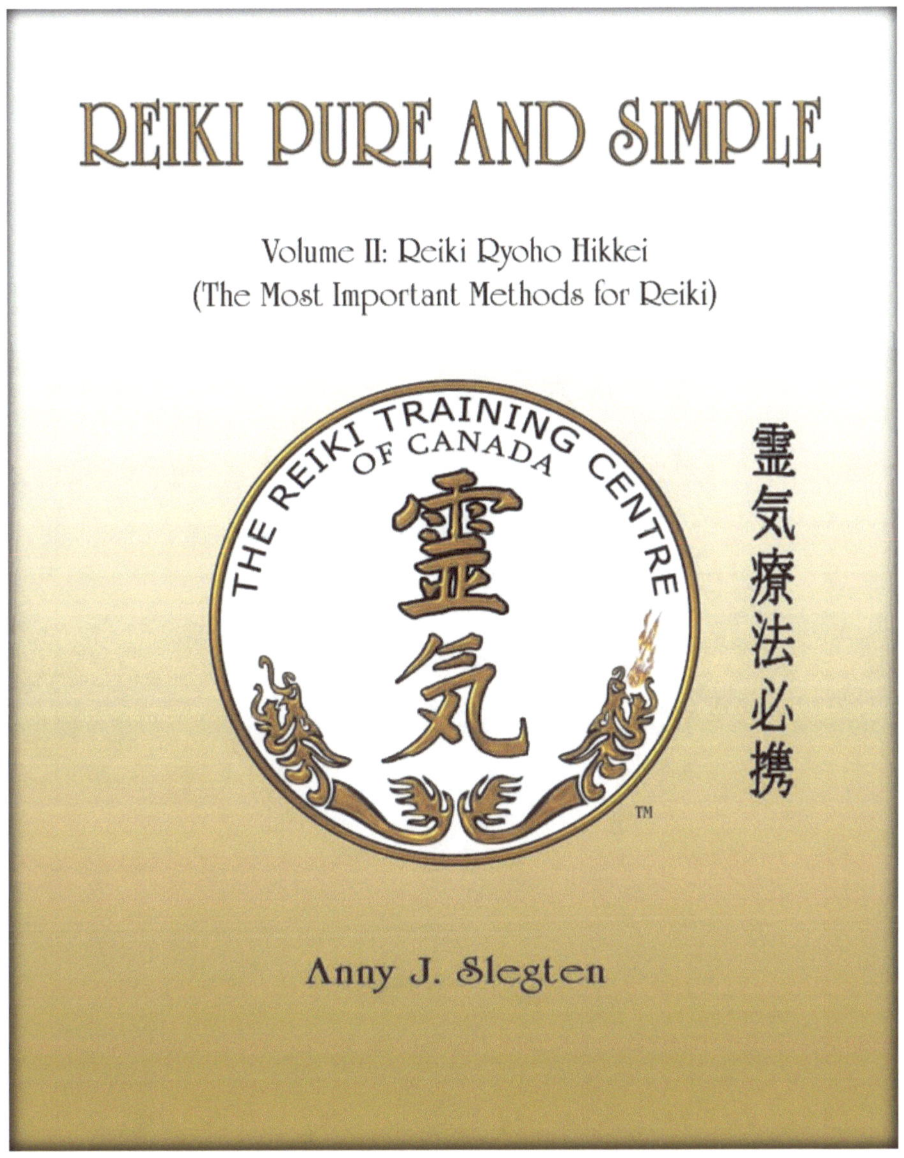

This book is a must read for Reiki Practitioners
regardless of their spiritual lineage
and could be of great benefit to Energy Healers
http://www.reiki-canada.com

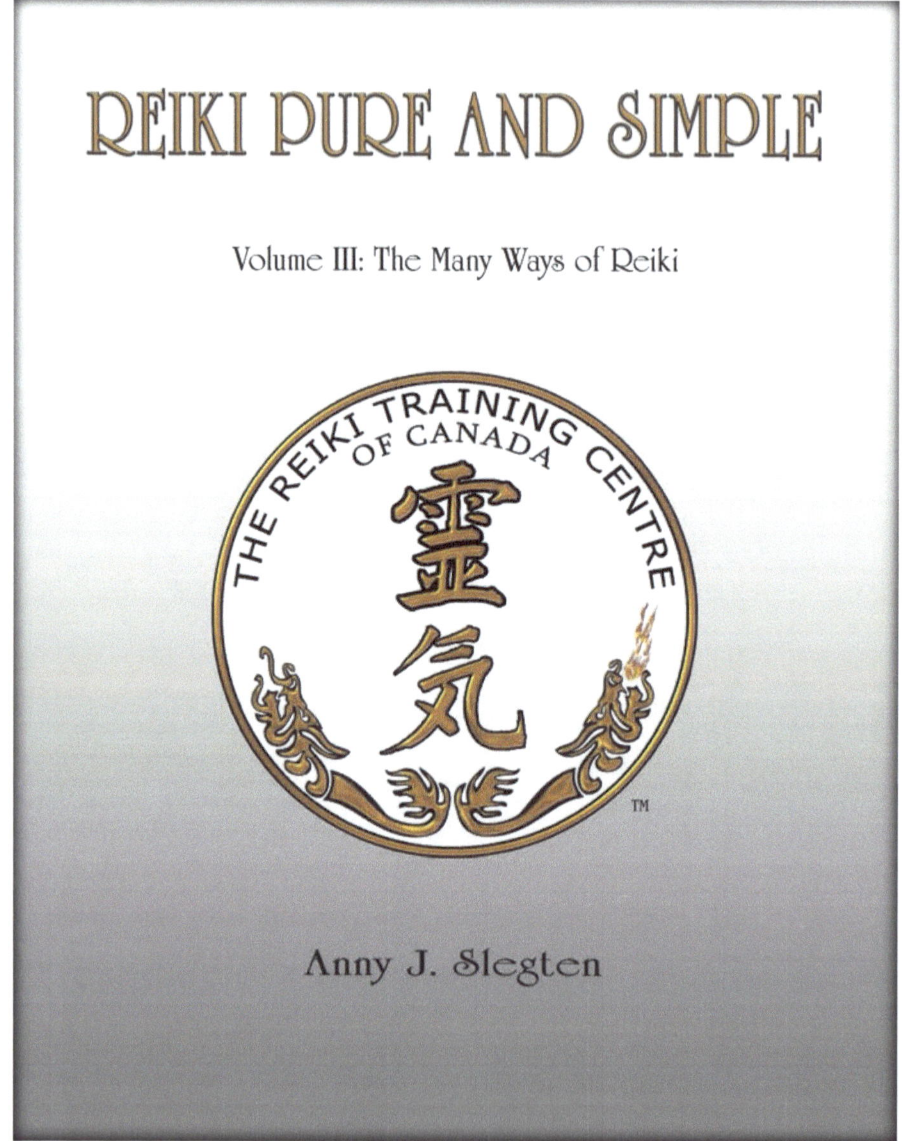

The Many Ways of Reiki
http://www.reiki-canada.com

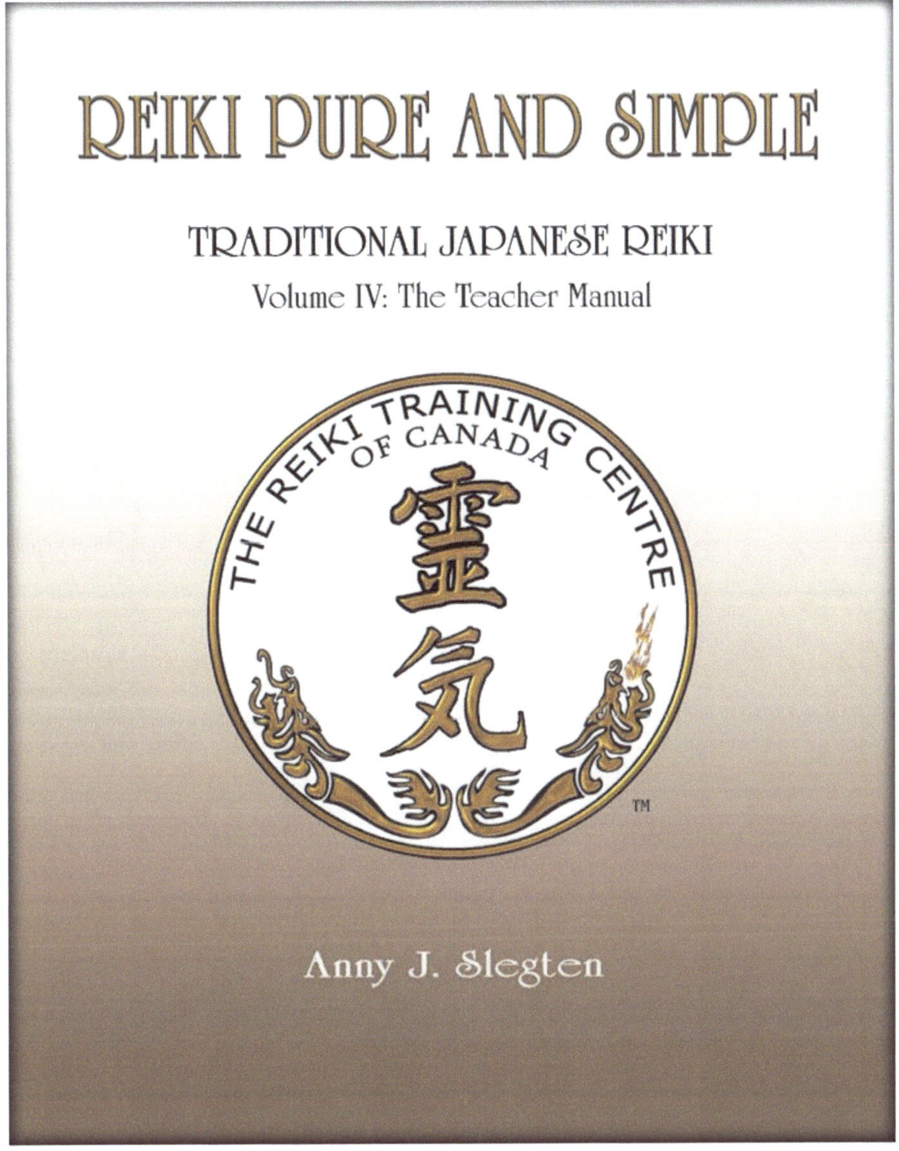

The Reiki Training Centre of Canada
Teacher's Manual
http://www.reiki-canada.com

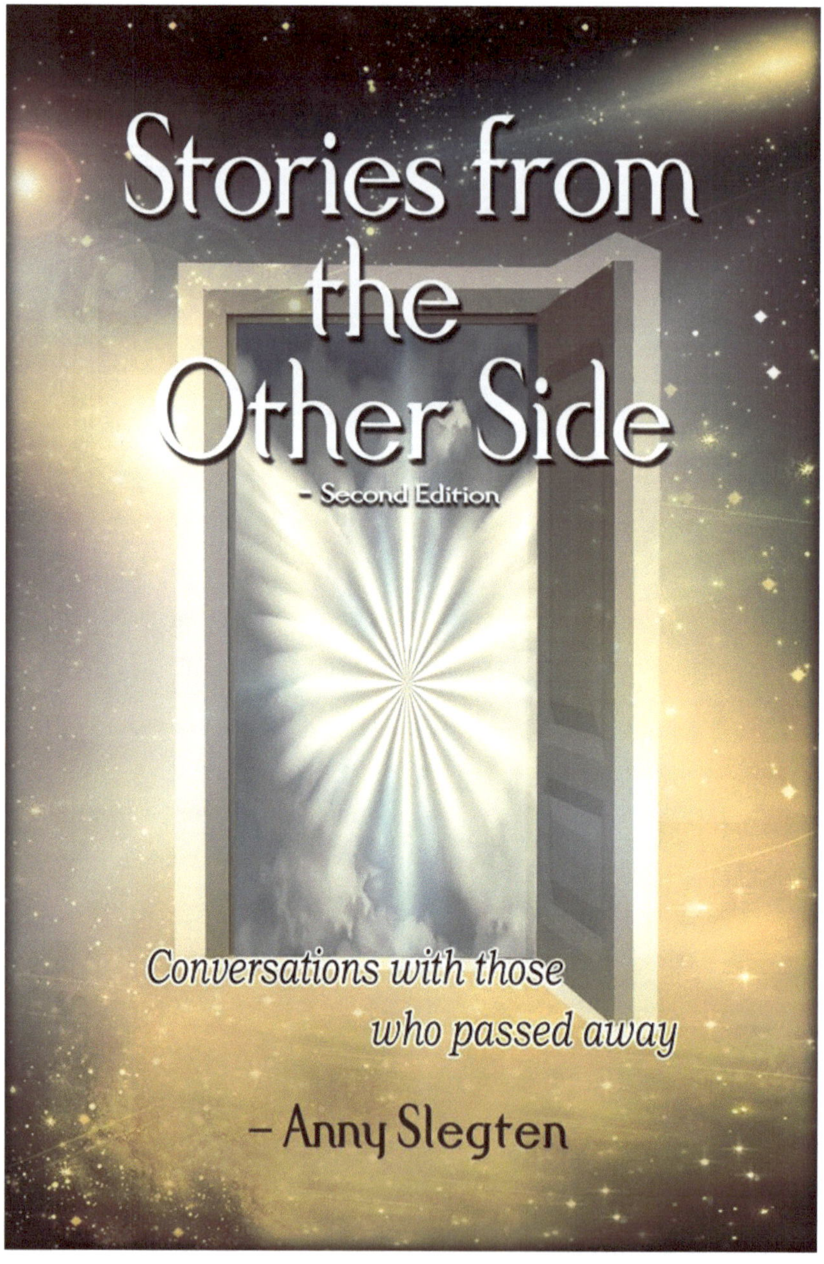

Stories from The Other Side – Second Edition
http://www.connectwithanny.com

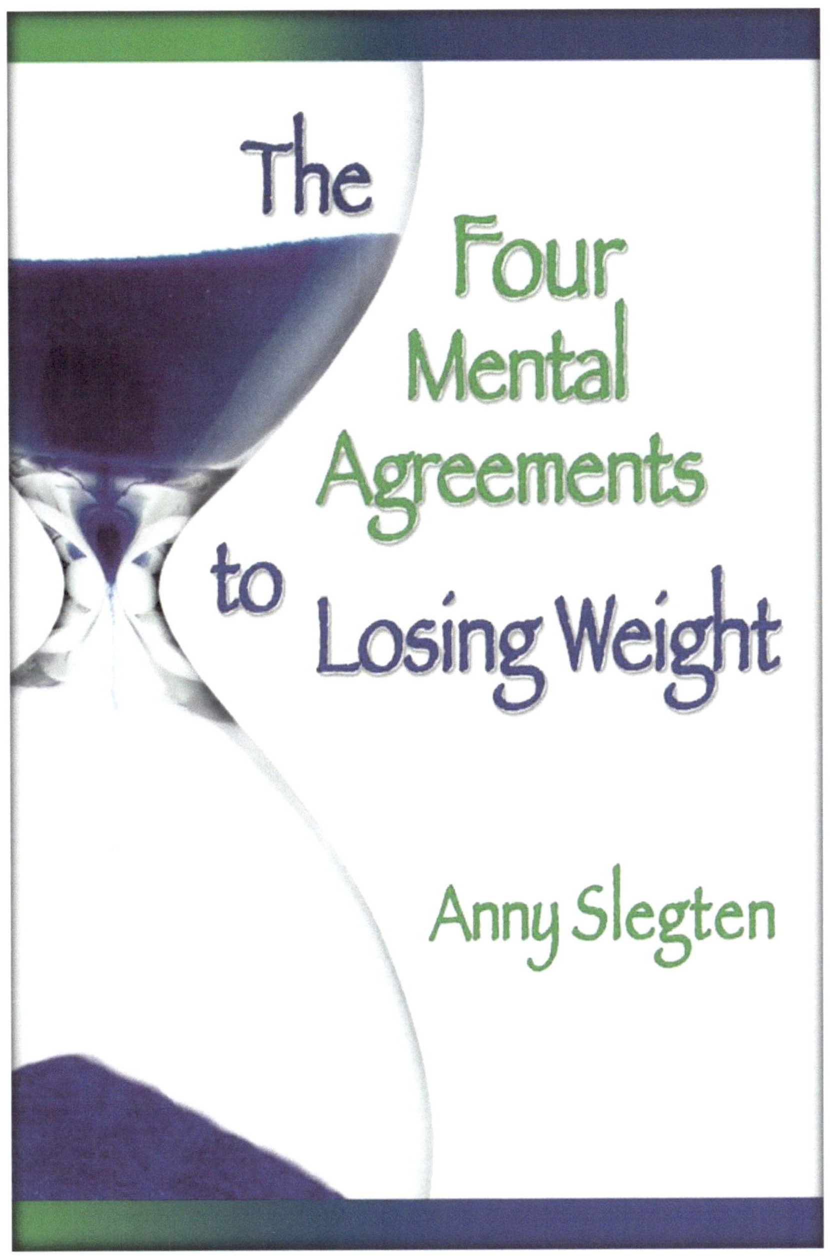

The Four Mental Agreements
To Losing Weight
http://www.connectwithanny.com

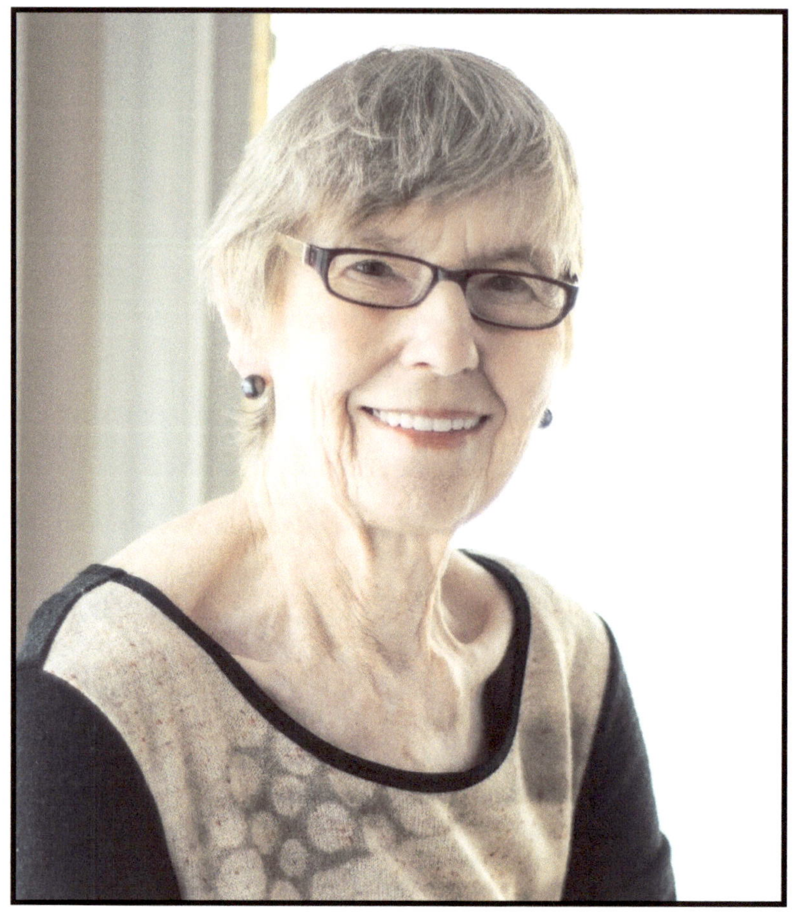

About The Author

As Director of The Hypnotism Training Institute of Alberta and The Reiki Training Centre of Canada, Anny has developed and structured the training and curriculum to the highest standards for both The Hypnotism Training Institute of Alberta and the Reiki Training Centre of Canada.

She offers training to students that come from all over Canada and around the world.

Anny has experienced and lived in many corners of the globe and this has given her a unique understanding of many cultures.

Anny's Belgian parents were from the Flemish part of Belgium and were speaking Flemish (Dutch) at home. Living in Congo, everything was in French.

Although she never spoke Flemish (Dutch), Anny speaks English with a guttural Dutch/German accent. Living in the English-speaking part of Canada for decades, Anny now speaks French with an English accent!

Anny is an Author and holds certifications as:

Master Hypnotist
Clinical Hypnotherapist
Hypno-Baby Birthing Facilitator and Instructor
HypnoBirthing™ Fertility Therapist for Men & Women
Reiki Master/Teacher
Master Remote Viewer

Anny is a world renowned Clinical Hypnotherapist and Hypnologist in full time practice since 1984 as well as a Hypno-Energy worker since 2008.

In 1986 Anny created and developed an unique method using hypnosis for distance services - Virtual Sessions.

Over the years these Virtual Sessions proved to be an effective, useful, and efficient method for investigations and putting closure on both present and past issues - resulting in peace of mind.

To know more about Anny, please visit www.annyslegten.com and make sure to read what she published on her Blog.

Do you wonder what else Anny is publishing?

Visit www.connectwithanny.com

www.ingramcontent.com/pod-product-compliance
Lightning Source LLC
LaVergne TN
LVHW070116110826
845147LV00002B/132

* 9 7 8 1 7 7 7 5 3 3 2 0 5 *